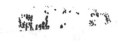

D0554130

BASICS OF
HEART FAILURE
A PROBLEM SOLVING APPROACH

August, 2019

To Sharp Chula Vista Library,

with best wishes.

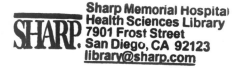
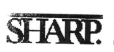

BASICS OF
HEART FAILURE
A PROBLEM SOLVING APPROACH

Brian E. Jaski, M.D.

Medical Director
Advanced Heart Failure and Cardiac Transplant Programs
Sharp Memorial Hospital
San Diego, CA

Associate Clinical Professor of Medicine
University of California, San Diego School of Medicine

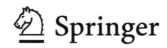 Springer

Author
Brian E. Jaski

ISBN-10: 0-7923-7786-9   ISBN-13: 978-0-7923-7786-3

Library of Congress Control Number: 00-020848

Printed on acid free paper

9 8 7 6 5 4

springer.com

For Cindy, K.C., and my parents.

Contents

Basics of Heart Failure

Part I — The Problem of Heart Failure

CHAPTER 4 — ORGAN

Part II: The Management of Heart Failure

CHAPTER 9 — DIAGNOSIS

Chapter 11 — Inpatient Therapy

Author's Note

The intent of this book is to provide a readable, concise guide that spans both the basis for clinical algorithms and the use of evidence based treatment guidelines. In part, this represents an outgrowth of a Heart Failure and Cardiac Transplant rotation at Sharp Memorial Hospital in San Diego for Balboa Navy cardiology fellows — now in its 10th year.

I am deeply indebted to many individuals. First is Joe Kim, presently pursuing a Ph.D. at the University of Minnesota Department of Epidemiology, who provided both technical expertise and steady optimism beginning over three years ago. Leigh Reardon and Susan Rademacher, who through their enthusiasm, intelligence, and hard work, reinforced my commitment to complete the project. Drs. Larry Deckelbaum and Len Lilly assisted me with their comments and advice. I thank Mr. Frank Wade for his support. The generosity of the Sharp Foundation helped develop this book from its inception. My colleagues and coworkers at the San Diego Cardiac Center and Sharp Memorial Hospital have been my clinical companions in caring for patients with heart failure over the past 15 years. Drs. Walter Abelmann, Patrick Serruys, and Sid Smith, by their examples, inspired me to want to write this book in the first place.

I hope that *Basics of Heart Failure* offers solutions to those caring for patients with heart failure — my efforts will then be justified.

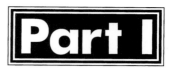

Introduction

A definition of heart failure depends on your perspective: as a clinician, a state of circulatory congestion; as an epidemiologist, an accelerating public health problem; as a physiologist, a decompensation of the circulation secondary to primary changes in the heart and subsequent changes in the vasculature; as a molecular biologist, a maladaptive response to biologic factors affecting the cardiac and vascular cell growth cycle; as a patient, a long-term disabling condition with uncertain survival.

Clinical Definition of Heart Failure

A syndrome including circulatory congestion or inadequate tissue perfusion, due to abnormal heart function and associated neurohormonal abnormalities.

In Part I, The Problem of Heart Failure, I ask you to view these perspectives as complementary. Often, helping a patient with heart failure begins with selecting the most appropriate initial frame of reference. For instance, whereas hemodynamics is a useful framework for *acute* heart failure, epidemiology and molecular biology may be more appropriate for *chronic* heart failure. By understanding the foundations and approaches to the problems of heart failure, you will be better prepared to understand and treat its many facets.

The spectrum of heart failure extends from the population to the molecule. Levels correspond with disciplines that together constitute the syndrome of heart failure.[1]

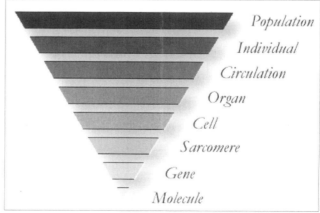

Population

Individual

Circulation

Organ

Cell

Sarcomere

Gene

Molecule

Figure i-i. *The spectrum of heart failure.*

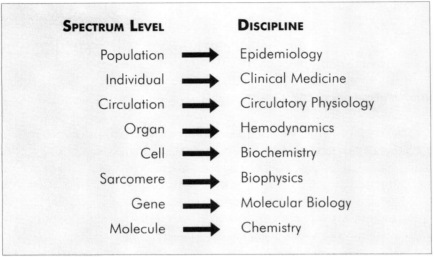

SPECTRUM LEVEL		DISCIPLINE
Population	➡	Epidemiology
Individual	➡	Clinical Medicine
Circulation	➡	Circulatory Physiology
Organ	➡	Hemodynamics
Cell	➡	Biochemistry
Sarcomere	➡	Biophysics
Gene	➡	Molecular Biology
Molecule	➡	Chemistry

Figure i-ii. *Helping a patient with heart failure often begins with selecting the most appropriate initial frame of reference.*

In Part II, The Management of Heart Failure, I outline a strategy for you to solve heart failure problems with the ultimate aim of helping patients feel better and live longer. This is no easy task; in part, because our knowledge base and tools are incomplete. In addition, to succeed you must gain the cooperation of your patients as active participants in their care since the management of heart failure can touch so many aspects of their lives.

Population

Chapter 1

Heart failure has profound public health implications. This chapter uses the perspective of the clinical epidemiologist to outline who has heart failure, the common etiologies of heart failure, and the medical costs associated with the care of these patients.

Incidence and Prevalence of Heart Failure

We live in an era of heart failure of epidemic proportions. In the United States, the incidence of heart failure increased from 250,000 to 400,000 new cases per year from 1970 to 1990.[1] Heart failure represents the cumulative outcome of all insults to the heart over time associated with changes in the peripheral vasculature. As patients survive manifestations of acute cardiovascular disease, late progression to heart failure becomes more common secondary to chronic ventricular enlargement and remodeling.[1-4]

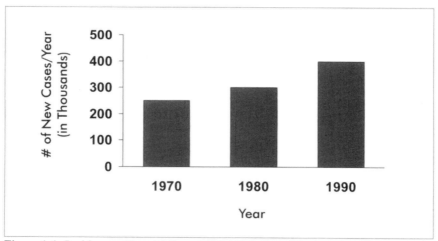

Figure 1-1. *Incidence of heart failure (1970-1990).* From The American Heart Association, *Heart and Stroke Facts*, 1998.[1]

☑ *About 4.8 million Americans have heart failure.*[1]

Similarly, it is not surprising that heart failure increases with age. The *prevalence* of heart failure approximately doubles with each decade of life.

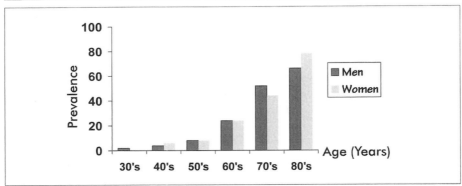

Figure 1-2. *Prevalence of heart failure per 1,000 population, by gender and age.* Reprinted with permission from The American College of Cardiology (Journal of the American College of Cardiology, October 1993:22:8A).[3]

In a community cross-sectional study of all patients with heart failure, 88% were greater than 65 years of age and 49% were older than 80 years of age.[5] Ten percent of individuals over the age of 80 have heart failure.

Death from Heart Failure

Because of the increasing incidence of heart failure, high age-specific death rates persist despite improved therapies.[6] High mortality associated with non-cardiac (for example, infection, neoplasia) or cardiac (for example, myocardial ischemia, arrhythmia) events may contribute to these findings. It is possible with greater use of therapies shown to improve survival, age-specific death rates will fall in the future.

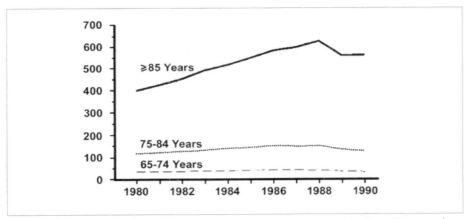

Figure 1-3. *Age-specific heart failure crude death rate for persons older than 65 years of age (per 100,000 population).* From the CDC, Morbidity and Mortality Weekly Report, 1994; 5:77-81.[6]

Total deaths from heart failure have risen over the last 30 years, due to the increasing age of the United States population and the increasing incidence of heart failure with age.

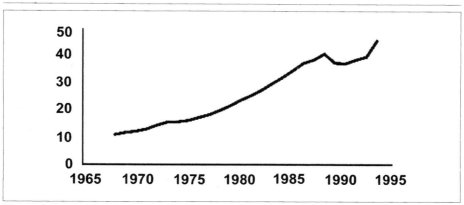

Figure 1-4. *Deaths from heart failure in thousands (years 1968 to 1993). Note: the decrease occurring in 1989 is attributed to a revision of the death certificate.* From the NIH; National Heart, Lung, and Blood Institute; CHF in the United States: A New Epidemic.[7]

Increase in Coronary Artery Disease (CAD) as Etiology of Heart Failure Over Four Decades

From 1950 to 1970, hypertension was the major etiology of heart failure. With improvements in the treatment of hypertension, atherosclerotic coronary artery disease is now a dominant cause of heart failure in the United States.[8] Frequently, multiple conditions contribute to heart failure.[9] Other etiologies of heart failure include cardiomyopathy and valvular heart disease. Valvular disease is important to identify because valve surgery often returns cardiac performance to normal.

☑ *Coronary artery disease and hypertension are the leading causes of heart failure. Cardiomyopathy and valvular heart disease are less frequent, but important etiologies of heart failure.*

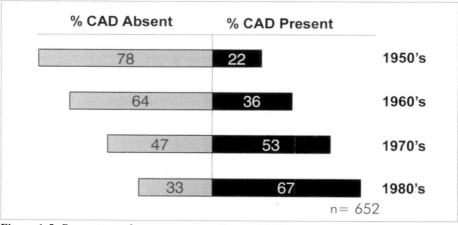

Figure 1-5. *Percentage of coronary artery disease (CAD) as the etiology for heart failure.*[9]

Hypertension and Heart Failure

Severity of hypertension predicts the occurrence of heart failure (Figure 1-6). Hypertension can lead to heart failure either on the basis of systolic dysfunction (low ejection fraction) or diastolic dysfunction (restricted filling of the heart). Increased peripheral resistance increases left ventricular work. Finally, high blood pressure is frequently a contributing factor to other etiologies of heart failure in patients who also have coronary artery disease, valvular heart disease or cardiomyopathy.[7] The recently released sixth report of the Joint National Committee on prevention, detection, evaluation, and treatment of high blood pressure recommends treating blood pressure to a goal of less than 140/90 mm Hg or lower in all individuals.[10] In patients with heart failure, however, a goal of less than 130/85 mm Hg is recommended.

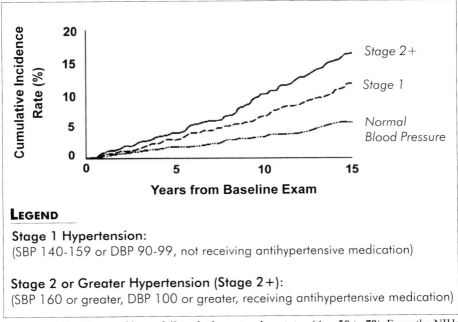

LEGEND

Stage 1 Hypertension:
(SBP 140-159 or DBP 90-99, not receiving antihypertensive medication)

Stage 2 or Greater Hypertension (Stage 2+):
(SBP 160 or greater, DBP 100 or greater, receiving antihypertensive medication)

Figure 1-6. *Incidence of heart failure by hypertension status (Age 50 to 79).* From the NIH; National Heart, Lung, and Blood Insititue; CHF in the United States: A New Epidemic.[7]

☑ *In patients with heart failure, a goal blood pressure of less than 130/85 mm Hg is recommended.*

Relationship Between Severity of Heart Failure and One-year Mortality

In patients with heart failure, mortality increases as functional status deteriorates. Functional status is commonly estimated by the New York Heart Association functional classification. Sudden death, defined as death occurring within one hour of the onset of worsening symptoms, accounts for approximately half of total mortality.[11] Since death in the most advanced patients is more frequently secondary to worsening heart failure, the remaining incidence of sudden death is less.[12]

NYHA Functional Class	Annual Mortality (%)[12]	Sudden Death (%)[12]
II	5-15	50-80
III	20-50	30-50
IV	30-70	5-30

NEW YORK HEART ASSOCIATION (NYHA) FUNCTIONAL CLASS

Class I: No limitation of functional activity.
Class II: Slight limitation of activity. Dyspnea and fatigue with moderate physical activity.
Class III: Marked limitation of activity. Dyspnea with minimal activity.
Class IV: Severe limitation of activity. Symptoms are present even at rest.

Etiology of Sudden Death

The mechanism of sudden death in patients with heart failure is important since medication and automatic defibrillator or pacemaker placement can potentially prevent deaths due to tachy- and brady- arrhythmias. Overall, ventricular tachyarrhythmias are the most common cause of sudden death in patients with left ventricular dysfunction.[11, 13] Other etiologies of circulatory collapse (for example, pulmonary embolism, myocardial infarction, sepsis, refractory pump dysfunction, or associated metabolic derangements) may also cause sudden death associated with bradycardic rhythms or pulseless electrical activity, especially in patients with the most advanced left ventricular dysfunction.[13]

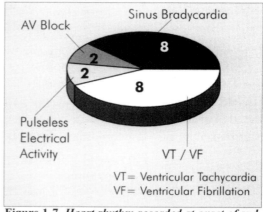

Figure 1-7. *Heart rhythm recorded at onset of sudden death in 20 patients with heart failure awaiting heart transplant.*[13]

Heart Failure in Men vs. Women
(Framingham, Massachusetts)

The Framingham Massachusetts Heart Data Base[3,4] found the annual incidence of heart failure in men to be almost twice that in women. In part, this reflects a greater incidence of ischemic disease and alcoholic cardiomyopathy in men. Women, however, are more likely to have diastolic dysfunction (65% in women versus 25% in men) — a less severe form of heart failure — that correlates to better survival.[14] Even in patients with severe systolic dysfunction, survival is better in women than men.[15] Thus, excluding patients who die rapidly after the diagnosis, the median survival in women is 2.2 years greater than in men. The greater survival and lower incidence of heart failure in women nets a similar *prevalence* of heart failure in both men and women.[4]

	MEN	WOMEN
Annual Incidence (Age >45)	7.2/1000	4.7/1000
Median Survival (excluding <90 day mortality)	3.2 years	5.4 years
Diabetes	14%	26%

Figure 1-8. *Heart failure in men vs. women.* [3]

☑ *Since 1946, the Framingham Heart Data Base has followed a cohort of 5192 patients and their offspring.*

Diabetes is a risk factor for the development of heart failure especially in women. This may be due to myocardial, metabolic, and microvascular changes induced by chronic hyperglycemia. Prior to the development of systolic dysfunction, diabetic patients may have a blunted increase of left ventricular contractility with exercise due to impairment of sympathetic innervation.[16]

The Economic Cost of Heart Failure

From1979 to 1992, hospital discharges including the diagnosis of heart failure more than doubled. Medicare hospital costs accounted for expenditures of $5.45 billion in 1991 with total medical costs of heart failure estimated at $38.1 billion annually.[17]

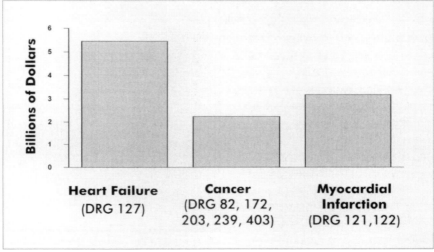

Figure 1-9. *Comparison of Heath Care Financing Administration (HCFA) expenditures of heart failure compared with cancer and myocardial infarction according to the Medicare program.* Reprinted with permission from Mosby, Inc.; O'Connell, JB; The Journal of Heart and Lung Transplantation; Economic Impact of Heart Failure in the United States: Time for a Different Approach. 1994; 13:S110.[17]

☑ *Heart Failure costs the United States an estimated $38.1 billion annually.*

Paul Dudley White

(1886-1973)

Paul Dudley White became known as the 'father of cardiology' in the United States. White was 27 years old when he traveled to England to study applications of the new electrocardiograph machine. The following year he returned to the Massachusetts General Hospital where he spent nearly 60 years of his life as a clinician. His use of the electrocardiogram included identifying arrhythmias and the clinical features of ventricular pre-excitation that became known as the Wolff-Parkinson-White syndrome. White promoted a clinical strategy of identifying the etiology, anatomy, physiology, functional status, and

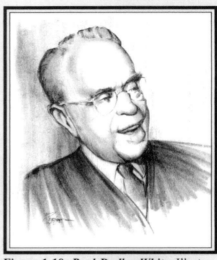

Figure 1-10. *Paul Dudley White.* Illustration by Peter Chapman.

prognosis in all cardiac patients. His goal was to understand the etiology of heart disease in part to aid in its eventual prevention. Clinical pearls that he taught included:[18]

"The most common cause of 'right heart' failure is 'left heart failure.'"
"Isolated left pleural fluid is not usually due to heart failure."

White promoted his personal philosophy for health of optimism, regular exercise (especially bicycling), and productive work. He published almost 600 scientific papers and 15 books during his career.

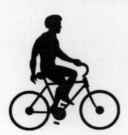

White advocated clinical observation, cardiovascular epidemiology, and clinical research. His compassionate care of countless patients inspired generations of emerging cardiologists.

Chapter 1 Quiz

1. Each year approximately _____ people have a new onset of heart failure in the US.
   a) 4,000
   b) 40,000
   c) 400,000
   d) 4,000,000

2. Due to recent advances in the treatment of cardiovascular disease, the age-related death rate of heart failure has significantly declined over the past decade.
   a) True
   b) False

3. From 1950 to 1970, _____ was the major etiology of heart failure. With improvements in the treatment of this etiologic factor, _____ is now the dominant cause of heart failure in the US.
   a) coronary artery disease; hypertension
   b) hypertension; coronary artery disease
   c) valvular disease; hypertension
   d) hypertension; valvular disease

4. The severity of hypertension predicts the occurrence of heart failure and can lead to heart failure on the basis of systolic or diastolic dysfunction.
   a) True
   b) False

5. Although the incidence of heart failure is greater in women than in men, men survive longer with heart failure, leading to a similar prevalence in any given age group of heart failure between men and women.
   a) True
   b) False

6. Heart failure costs the US an estimated _____ dollars annually.
   a) 38 million
   b) 380 million
   c) 38 billion
   d) 380 billion

See Appendix for solutions.

Individual

Chapter 2

Clinical medicine engages heart failure at the level of the individual. This chapter considers the presentations of heart failure and clinical tools that enable patient evaluation. Greater attention to clinical presentations and tools can be found in Chapter 9, Diagnosis.

Presentations of Heart Failure

Although heart failure may have protean manifestations, two characteristic presentations are useful to describe because patient objectives and priorities will differ based on the type of presentation.

DECOMPENSATED HEART FAILURE

Acute left heart failure of new onset can present with pulmonary edema. An aggressive and urgent approach is necessary to determine the etiology of heart failure. Early intervention may be important particularly in acute ischemic syndromes that can affect long-term outcome.

In a patient with a history of heart failure who presents in a decompensated state, your priority is less on diagnosis of the *etiology* of heart failure (this is usually known) and more on identification of *precipitating factors* and rapid treatment. A patient may have pulmonary edema, systemic congestion, or both. Alternatively, findings of low cardiac output presenting as fatigue, poor mentation, hypotension, and hepatic and renal dysfunction may predominate.

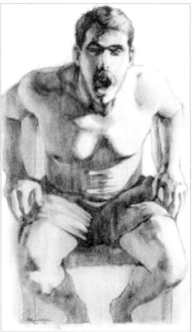

Figure 2-1. *Decompensated heart failure.* Illustration by Peter Chapman.

COMPENSATED CHRONIC HEART FAILURE

The patient with compensated heart failure represents a larger group of individuals. A patient may have either newly recognized or known chronic left ventricular dysfunction without overt decompensation. Symptoms of compensated heart failure, however, are often present with activity.

The patient treatment objectives for those with compensated heart failure differ from those for patients with decompensated heart failure. After treating causes of left ventricular dysfunction, the priority may be to delay or reverse disease progression by blunting cardiac structural change and enlargement over time.

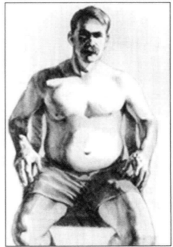

Figure 2-2. *Compensated heart failure.* Illustration by Peter Chapman.

Forward vs. Backward Heart Failure

Classification of forward versus backward heart failure relates a patient's abnormal clinical findings to either inadequate tissue perfusion or circulatory congestion, respectively. This has therapeutic implications since a state of inadequate perfusion, forward heart failure, may improve with an increase in circulating blood volume (increased salt and fluid intake or reduced diuretic therapy) whereas congestion, backward failure, requires a decrease in circulating blood volume (decreased salt and fluid intake or increased diuretic therapy). Vasodilator therapy may improve both, but can precipitate hypotension.

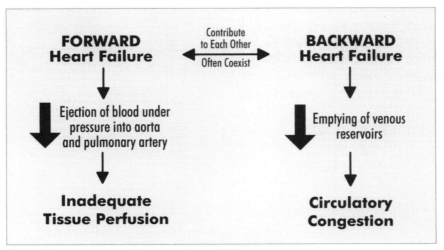

Figure 2-3. *Forward and backward heart failure.*

CLINICAL MANIFESTATIONS

A decompensated patient often may have *both* forward and backward heart failure. Inadequate tissue perfusion can lead to congestion through increased renal retention of salt and water along with reflex increased venous tone. Circulatory congestion can lead to a decrease in cardiac output through increased pulmonary artery pressure reducing right heart stroke volume and reflex increased arterial resistance to left heart ejection.

Useful Definitions

PULMONARY EDEMA

Accumulation of an excessive amount of fluid in the lungs, usually resulting from left ventricular failure.

DYSPNEA

Shortness of breath, a subjective difficulty or distress in breathing, usually associated with disease of the heart or lungs.

ORTHOPNEA

Difficulty in breathing which is brought on or aggravated by lying flat.

PAROXYSMAL NOCTURNAL DYSPNEA (PND)

Dyspnea which appears suddenly at night, usually waking the patient after an hour or two of sleep; caused by pulmonary congestion and edema which results from left sided heart failure.

CHEYNE-STOKES BREATHING

A pattern of breathing with a gradual increase in depth and sometimes in rate to a maximum, followed by a decrease resulting in apnea; the cycles ordinarily are 30 seconds to 2 minutes in duration, with 5 to 30 seconds of apnea. Related to the loss of feedback control of respiration in heart failure.

S_3 GALLOP

An additional heart sound after aortic and pulmonary valve closure (S_2) audible during early rapid filling of the left ventricle when left atrial pressure is increased.

Samuel Levine
(1891-1966)

Observations of a Senior Clinician On Detecting the Onset of Heart Failure

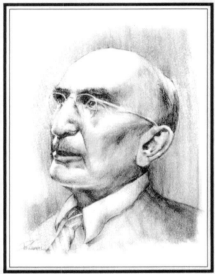

Figure 2-4. *Samuel Levine.* Illustration by Peter Chapman.

"Symptoms as a rule precede signs. Breathlessness is the most important and generally the earliest evidence of heart failure... it is necessary to rule out other causes, such as those of a functional and pulmonary nature, before regarding breathlessness as due entirely to the heart. In hypertension, aortic and coronary cases dyspnea may first appear at night, while in other cases it is first noted on effort. Cheyne-Stokes breathing especially during sleep almost always means heart failure. Even before dyspnea occurs most cardiac patients complain of fatigue, 'lack of pep,' restlessness, insomnia and nervousness."[1]

— **Samuel Levine, M.D.**
From *Clinical Heart Disease*, 1951

Left vs. Right Sided Heart Failure

Similar to forward versus backward heart failure, left versus right sided heart failure is a classification of clinical findings that also may occur together. Initially, isolated left heart failure (for example, caused by coronary artery disease) can lead to right heart failure because pulmonary congestion leads to an increase in pulmonary artery pressure that can affect right ventricular performance. Because ischemic, hypertensive, and valvular heart disease primarily affect left ventricular performance, left heart failure is a more common presenting clinical problem.

☑ *Left heart failure is more common than right heart failure.*

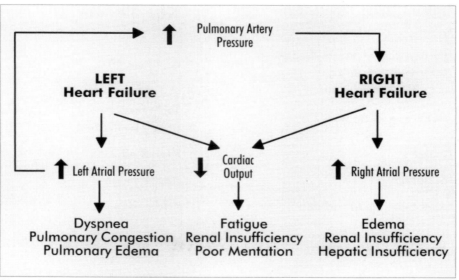

Figure 2-5. *Left and right heart failure.*

Clinical Criteria for Heart Failure

Data from the history, physical exam, or laboratory (for example, chest x-ray) may lead to the diagnosis of heart failure. Any one of the findings below can be the first clue to look for underlying left or right ventricular dysfunction. In general, clinical heart failure is present when evidence of left or right ventricular dysfunction is present with associated patient symptoms.[2]

☑ *Heart failure = Cardiac Dysfunction + Symptoms*

Major Criteria	Minor Criteria
Acute pulmonary edema	Dyspnea on exertion
Paroxysmal nocturnal dyspnea or orthopnea response	Night cough
Neck-vein distention	Tachycardia (>120 beats/min)
Rales	Pleural effusion
S_3 gallop	Hepatomegaly
Abdominojugular reflux	Ankle edema
Cardiomegaly on CXR	Vital capacity decrease (1/3 from max)
Increased venous pressure (> 16cm H_2O)	
Weight loss >4.5kg 5 days into treatment can be classified as a major or minor criterion	

Figure 2-6. *The diagnosis of heart failure, in the Framingham heart failure study, requires two major or one major and two minor criteria to be present concurrently. Minor criteria cannot be attributed to another medical condition.*[2]

Cardiac Presentations in Patients with Heart Failure

When a patient with a history of heart failure develops an acute worsening of symptoms, you have to determine if the problem is cardiac or non-cardiac. If cardiac, it may be due to worsening heart failure, myocardial ischemia, or arrhythmia.

Multiple cardiac findings may present together because of the balance maintained by the stable patient with heart failure prior to deterioration. Effective intervention can depend on identifying the *primary* reason for decompensation and initiating prompt treatment.

☑ *Worsening heart failure, myocardial ischemia, and arrhythmias can present together.*

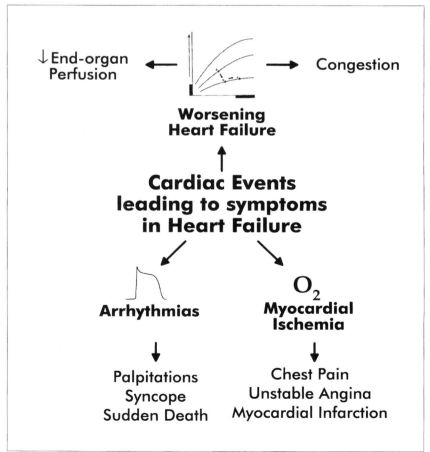

Figure 2-7. *Cardiac presentations in patients with heart failure.*

Predictive Value of Clinical Findings for Estimating Hemodynamics in Heart Failure

Drs. Lynn Stevenson and Joe Perloff evaluated the sensitivity and specificity of a range of clinical factors to predict the findings of right heart catheterization in 50 patients *with known chronic heart failure* being evaluated for heart transplant. The presence or absence of a recent history of shortness of breath while patients were supine requiring extra pillows (orthopnea) was the most predictive factor of a pulmonary capillary wedge pressure being either elevated (greater than 22 mm Hg)

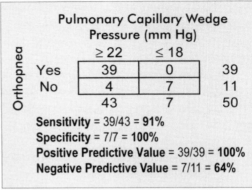

		Pulmonary Capillary Wedge Pressure (mm Hg)		
		≥ 22	≤ 18	
Orthopnea	Yes	39	0	39
	No	4	7	11
		43	7	50

Sensitivity = 39/43 = **91%**
Specificity = 7/7 = **100%**
Positive Predictive Value = 39/39 = **100%**
Negative Predictive Value = 7/11 = **64%**

Figure 2-8. *Orthopnea was a more sensitive predictor of wedge pressure than other history or physical exam findings in patients with known advanced heart failure.*[3]

or less than 18 mm Hg. None of their patients had a wedge pressure between these two values.[3]

Physical exam findings of congestion were relatively *insensitive* to detect an elevated pulmonary capillary wedge pressure. Peripheral edema, neck vein distention, or rales were present in only 50% of patients with a high wedge pressure. When any of these findings were present on physical exam, however, it was *specific* for a pulmonary capillary wedge pressure of greater than 22 mm Hg.

PROPORTIONAL PULSE PRESSURE AND HEART FAILURE

In general, arterial pulse pressure is proportional to left ventricular stroke volume. Stevenson and Perloff also found that a proportional pulse pressure (pulse pressure divided by the systolic pressure) less than 25% was the best discriminator for predicting a low cardiac index (< 2.2 L/min/m²). This measure had a high positive and negative predictive value for identifying normal versus depressed cardiac index. Proportional pulse pressure and cardiac index also correlated in a linear relationship over a range of values.

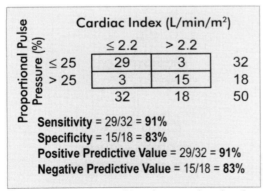

		Cardiac Index (L/min/m²)		
		≤ 2.2	> 2.2	
Proportional Pulse Pressure (%)	≤ 25	29	3	32
	> 25	3	15	18
		32	18	50

Sensitivity = 29/32 = **91%**
Specificity = 15/18 = **83%**
Positive Predictive Value = 29/32 = **91%**
Negative Predictive Value = 15/18 = **83%**

Figure 2-9. *Relationship of proportional pulse pressure and cardiac index in 50 patients with heart failure.*[3]

Use of Inducible Abdominojugular Reflux to Increase Sensitivity of Physical Exam in Heart Failure

Although patients with elevated pulmonary capillary wedge pressures (see previous section) may not have elevated jugular venous distention at rest, sensitivity is improved when combined with bedside inducible jugular venous distention achieved by examining neck veins while compressing the patient's abdomen (abdominojugular reflux or hepatojugular reflux). Butman and co-workers defined a positive test as internal or external jugular vein distention when applying manual abdominal pressure in the center of the patient's upper abdomen for 10 seconds with release leading to an abrupt fall greater than or equal to 4 cm.[4]

Nine of 16 patients with chronic heart failure and pulmonary capillary wedge pressure greater than 18 mm Hg had a positive abdominojugular reflux in the *absence* of resting jugular venous distention.

Abdominojugular Reflux (AJR)
Pulmonary Capillary Wedge Pressure (mm Hg)

	> 18	≤ 18	
+ JVD or +AJR	30	3	33
- JVD and -AJR	7	12	19
	37	15	52

Sensitivity = 30/37 = **81%**
Specificity = 12/15 = **80%**
PPV = 30/33 = **91%**
NPV = 12/19 = **63%**

Jugular Venous Distension (JVD)
Pulmonary Capillary Wedge Pressure (mm Hg)

Jugular Venous Distension		> 18	≤ 18	
	+	21	1	22
	-	16	14	30
		37	15	52

Sensitivity = 21/37 = **57%**
Specificity = 14/15 = **93%**
PPV = 21/22 = **95%**
NPV = 14/30 = **47%**

PPV — Positive Predictive Value
NPV — Negative Predictive Value

Figure 2-10. *Jugular venous distension, (with or without a positive abdominojugular reflux test) and pulmonary wedge pressure.*[4]

Chapter 2 Quiz

1. Paroxysmal nocturnal dyspnea is usually described as:

    a) a pattern of breathing with a gradual increase in depth and sometimes in rate to a maximum, followed by a decrease resulting in apnea

    b) discomfort in breathing which is brought on or aggravated by lying flat

    c) dyspnea which appears suddenly at night, usually waking the patient after an hour or two of sleep

    d) none of the above

2. Complete this analogy: Forward heart failure: Inadequate tissue perfusion :: Backward heart failure: _____

    a) Pulmonary congestion

    b) Hypertension

    c) Coronary artery disease

    d) None of the above

3. Some common manifestations of left heart failure include dyspnea, pulmonary congestion, and pulmonary edema. Right heart failure usually leads to:

    a) edema, abdominal pain, and hepatic insufficiency

    b) dyspnea, pulmonary edema, and pulmonary insufficiency

    c) edema, pulmonary and renal insufficiency

    d) none of the above

4. According to the Framingham Heart Study, all of the following are considered a 'major' criteria for heart failure except:

    a) night cough

    b) acute pulmonary edema

    c) S_3 gallop

    d) neck-vein distention

5. All of the following cardiac events lead to an increase in symptoms in the patients with heart failure <u>except</u>:

    a) arrhythmias

    b) myocardial ischemia

    c) absent abdominojugular reflux

    d) worsening heart failure

6. In patients with known advanced heart failure, orthopnea was a more sensitive predictor of pulmonary capillary wedge pressure than other history or physical exam findings.

    a) True

    b) False

7. In the patient with chronic heart failure, a physical exam can be free of findings of lung congestion despite a markedly elevated pulmonary capillary wedge pressure.

    a) True

    b) False

See Appendix for solutions.

Circulation

Chapter 3

Normal cardiac function relies on the actions of circulatory mechanisms and controls. In this chapter, circulatory physiology is examined with the aim of elucidating models of heart failure, pinpointing targets of therapy, and identifying neurohormonal mediators of the progression of heart failure.

Block Diagram of Circulation

In general, the closed loop circulation allows measurement of blood flow at any central point to determine output from the right and left ventricles or through the pulmonary and systemic circulations. Inflow and outflow valves within each ventricle maintain the uni-directional flow of blood.

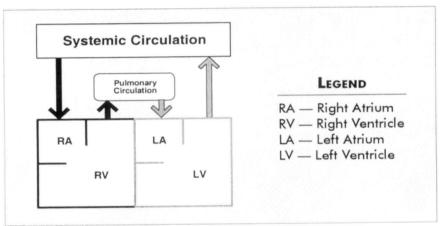

Figure 3-1. *Circulatory block diagram of the heart.*

Normal and Heart Failure Hemodynamics

Hemodynamic status can be estimated based on history, physical exam, or non-invasive lab testing findings (see Chapter 2, Individual) or measured directly at the time of cardiac catheterization. By definition, acute or chronic *decompensated* heart failure is present when symptoms at rest are due to high filling pressures and/or depressed cardiac index. Blood pressure can be high, normal, or low depending, in part, on the systemic vascular resistance. A patient with a low ejection fraction may exhibit either normal or abnormal hemodynamics at rest in part depending on vascular tone and volume.

A patient with heart failure can have a markedly elevated right atrial pressure (for example, 16 mm Hg) secondary to decreased right ventricular function, increased venous tone due to increased neurohormonal activation, or increased total vascular volume due to increased renal retention of sodium and water.

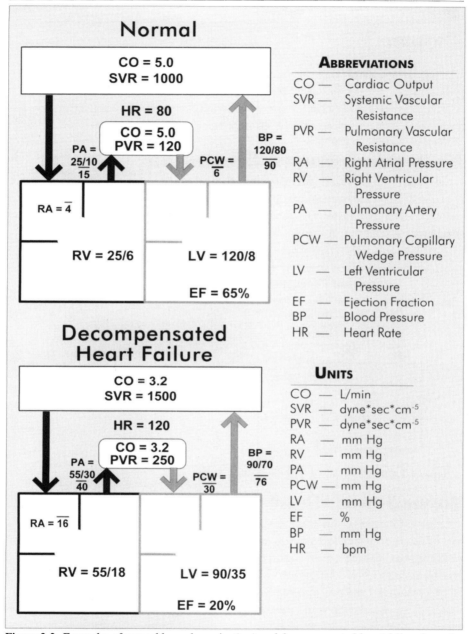

Figure 3-2. *Examples of normal hemodynamics (top) and decompenasted heart failure hemody-namics (bottom).*

☑ *Pulmonary capillary wedge pressure estimates left atrial pressure by floating a balloon tipped catheter from a central vein through the right heart to the pulmonary artery.*

Heart Failure Reduces Peak Oxygen Consumption with Exercise

Impairment with activity is the hallmark of symptoms of heart failure. Reasons for a reduced peak oxygen consumption with exercise include impaired augmentation of cardiac output (heart rate x stroke volume), pulmonary congestion, or skeletal muscle deconditioning.

OXYGEN CONSUMPTION

Oxygen consumption equals the difference between oxygen content delivery to the body (cardiac output x arterial oxygen concentration) minus oxygen content remaining when blood flow converges back to the central venous circulation (cardiac output x mixed venous or pulmonary artery oxygen concentration).

NORMAL RESPONSE TO EXERCISE IN A TRAINED INDIVIDUAL

A trained young individual can increase oxygen consumption 18-fold with exercise. This is achieved as a result of a threefold increase in heart rate (HR), a twofold increase in stroke volume (SV), and a threefold increase in tissue oxygen extraction — defined as the difference between arterial and venous blood oxygen concentration, ΔAVO_2.[1]

$$O_2 \text{ CONSUMPTION} = HR \times SV \times \Delta AVO_2$$

☑ *In a trained athlete, oxygen consumption may increase up to 18-fold with exercise.*

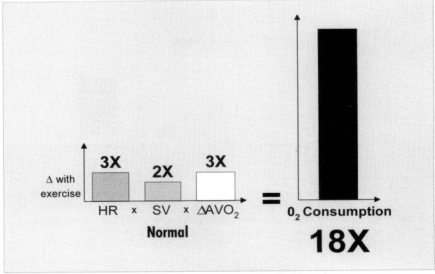

Figure 3-3. *Oxygen utilization with exercise in trained athletes.*[1]

HEART FAILURE RESPONSE TO EXERCISE

Compared with a normal individual, a patient with heart failure and an impaired increase of cardiac output with activity may have a fixed stroke volume and an increased resting heart rate. This could result in a blunted sixfold maximum potential increase in oxygen consumption with exercise when tissue extraction of oxygen (ΔAVO_2) can no longer increase.

☑ *Different mechanisms may lead to a reduced oxygen consumption with exercise.*

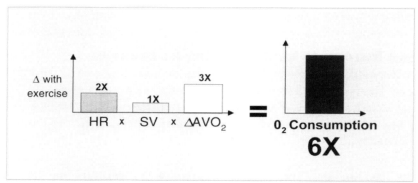

Figure 3-4. *Example of cardiac output limiting oxygen utilization with exercise in heart failure patients.*

Alternatively, a patient with heart failure and either symptoms of pulmonary congestion or skeletal muscle deconditioning will stop exercise before achieving a maximum tissue extraction of oxygen ($\Delta AVO_2 = 2x$).

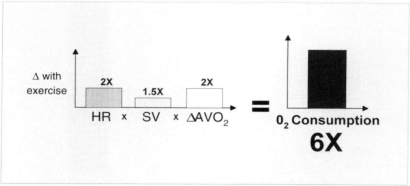

Figure 3-5. *Example of oxygen utilization limited by pulmonary congestion or skeletal muscle deconditioning in heart failure patients with exercise.*

Useful Definitions

AFTERLOAD
>   Ventricular pressure and volume *after the onset of contraction* that determine *sarcomere* shortening and, therefore, the resistance that the ventricle must overcome to eject its contents.

PRELOAD
>   Ventricular *end-diastolic* pressure and volume that determine resting *sarcomere* length *just prior to contraction.*

CONTRACTILITY (INOTROPIC STATE)
>   The intrinsic ability of the left or right ventricle to perform pressure-volume work as a pump *independent* of changes in preload or afterload.

☑   *Afterload affects performance throughout the duration of ventricular ejection while preload affects performance based on filling at the end of diastole.*

Ventricular Pressure-Volume Relationships

The right and left ventricles are phasic circulatory pumps that convert biochemical energy into mechanical pressure-volume work. Ejected stroke volume (SV) with each beat is the difference between end-diastolic and end-systolic volumes (Volume 1 – Volume 3).

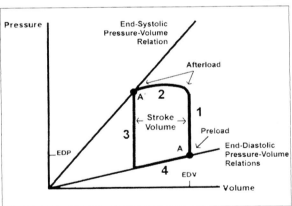

Figure 3-6. Phases of the cardiac cycle which occur with each heart beat. (1) Isovolumic systole, (2) Systolic ejection, (3) Isovolumic relaxation, (4) Diastolic filling.

EJECTION AND FILLING

Ejection fraction (EF) is the ratio of ejected stroke volume to end-diastolic volume (EDV). Ejection occurs against a hemodynamic arterial impedance to reach a point at end-systole defined by the characteristic end-systolic pressure-volume relation (normal EF = 55-75%). Filling from venous return in diastole occurs to a point defined by the end-diastolic pressure-volume relation (see page 56).

Useful Definitions

VASCULAR RESISTANCE

The ratio, R, of the mean pressure difference to the flow through a circulatory network.

Resistance = $\Delta P/C.O.$

Mean Systemic Vascular Resistance = $(\overline{Art}-\overline{RA})/C.O.$

Mean Pulmonary Vascular Resistance = $(\overline{PA}-\overline{PCW})/C.O.$

(see Appendix, page 273)

VASCULAR CAPACITANCE

The ratio of a change in fluid pressure distending a vascular segment to a change of volume within a segment.

Aortic Capacitance = (SBP-DBP)/SV

(see Appendix, page 273)

VASCULAR TONE

The elastic properties of venous and arterial vessels that determine their diameter, and thus, both their vascular resistance (Δ longitudinal pressure/flow) and capacitance (Δ vascular volume/ Δ transmural pressure).

Abbreviations

P —	Pressure	PA —	Pulmonary Artery Pressure
C.O. —	Cardiac Output	PCW —	Pulmonary Capillary
SVR —	Systemic Vascular Resistance		Wedge Pressure
Art —	Arterial Pressure	SBP —	Systolic Blood Pressure
RA —	Right Atrial Pressure	DBP —	Diastolic Blood Pressure
PVR —	Pulmonary Vascular Resistance	SV —	Stroke Volume

Vascular Tone Affects Ventricular Afterload and Preload

Vascular tone is a property of both veins and arteries. It is a composite of the collagen, elastin, and active smooth muscle cell properties of the vessel wall. Contraction of smooth muscle cells in a circumferential orientation within vascular walls reduces vessel diameter.

Physiologic or pharmacologic changes in vascular tone lead to similar effects on both arterial and venous smooth muscle contraction. For example, increased sympathetic tone causes vasoconstriction of both arteries and veins.

You cannot directly measure vascular tone even though it is an important physiological variable. Changes in arterial or venous vascular resistance or capacitance *imply* changes in vascular tone.

Arterial impedance or opposition to ejection from the left or right ventricle affects ventricular afterload. There is no universal measure of impedance or afterload, but you can estimate it by the systolic or mean arterial pressure or by the calculated vascular resistance. Functionally, vascular tone determines both arterial capacitance ($\Delta V/\Delta P$ transmural) and resistance (ΔP longitudinal/Flow).

PRELOAD

Venous capacitance and blood volume affect venous pressure, ventricular diastolic pressure, and preload.

☑ *Increased vascular tone increases arterial resistance and decreases arterial and venous capacitance.*

Site of Vascular Smooth Muscle	Functional Effect	Effect on Ventricular Load	Effect on Hemodynamics
↑ arterial tone	↑ systemic vascular resistance	↑ LV *afterload*	↑ mean arterial blood pressure
↑ aortic and large artery tone	↓ arterial capacitance	↑ LV *afterload*	↑ arterial pulse pressure
↑ venous tone	↓ venous capacitance	↑ RV and LV *preload*	↑ right atrial, pulmonary capillary wedge, and ventricular end-diastolic pressures

Figure 3-7. *The impact of vascular tone on circulation.*

The Frank-Starling Curve

The Frank-Starling Law of the Heart (Otto Frank, 1865-1944 and Ernest Starling, 1866-1927) states that increased heart filling leads to increased heart ejection of blood. This principle regulates the beat to beat control of the heart stroke volume to meet changes in circulatory conditions. Because of this property, heart size remains relatively stable despite variations in returning venous blood flow. Phasic differences between the right and left ventricular output balance to be, on average, equal.

PLOT OF FRANK-STARLING CURVE

A plot of stroke volume or cardiac output on the vertical axis versus left ventricular filling volume (preload) or end-diastolic pressure on the horizontal axis depicts this Law over a range of diastolic filling (Figure 3-8). Normal left ventricular function at rest or with exercise implies adequate tissue perfusion with ventricular filling pressures less than those associated with pulmonary congestion (a). Heart failure of any etiology can result in a downward shift of this curve and an operating point (b,c) associated with inadequate perfusion, pulmonary congestion, or both.

> ☑ *A "flat" Frank-Starling curve implies that increases in heart filling no longer lead to increases in cardiac output.*

BIOPHYSICAL MECHANISM

The basis for the Frank-Starling Law is multifactorial. Myocyte cell length (preload) affects actin and myosin overlap, crossbridge number, and intracellular calcium concentration that determines myocyte force and shortening (see Chapter 6, Sarcomere).[2]

Heart Failure and Afterload

For any given end-diastolic volume, a change in ejection performance or stroke volume can result from *either* a change in contractility or afterload. For example, following a myocardial infarction, a decrease in left ventricular performance could be secondary to either a decrease in contractility due to the loss of functioning myocytes, an increase in systemic vascular resistance, or both.

THERAPEUTIC IMPLICATIONS

You can improve the performance of the failing heart by either increasing contractility or decreasing afterload. However, a drug that increases contractility will increase myocardial oxygen consumption whereas a drug that reduces afterload will decrease myocardial oxygen consumption. Ultimately, systemic hypotension (low blood pressure) will limit improvements in ventricular performance achievable by afterload reduction alone.

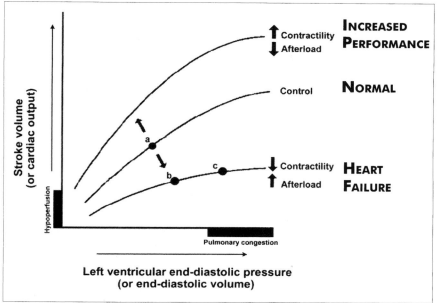

Figure 3-8. *The Frank-Starling left ventricular performance curves demonstrates that performance of a failing heart can improve with either an increase in contractility or a decrease in afterload. Normal LV function (a) is associated with adequate tissue perfusion without pulmonary congestion. Heart failure results in a downward shift of the curve resulting in hypoperfusion (b), pulmonary congestion (c), or both.*

☑ *Ultimately, hypotension limits acute improvements in ventricular performance with vasodilators alone.*

Relationships among Physiologic, Clinical, and Ventricular Function Variables

Three types of circulatory variables are relevant when caring for a patient with heart failure:

1. PHYSIOLOGIC VARIABLES
(VASCULAR TONE, INOTROPIC STATE/HEART RATE, BLOOD VOLUME)

Physiologic variables help us understand primary changes in the circulation based on pathophysiologic mechanisms. For example, vasoconstricting hormones (angiotensin II) or drugs (high dose dopamine) increase venous and arterial *Vascular Tone,* and therefore, increase both ventricular preload and afterload. Other physiologic variables affected by disease therapies are *Inotropic State* (with associated *Heart Rate*) and circulating *Blood Volume*.

2. CLINICAL VARIABLES
(BLOOD PRESSURE, CARDIAC OUTPUT/HEART RATE, FILLING PRESSURES)

Clinical variables may be directly measured from a patient and are affected by changes in physiologic variables. Acute changes in clinically measured variables imply changes in physiologic variables. Clinical variables include *Blood Pressure, Cardiac Output* and right and left ventricular *Filling Pressures.*

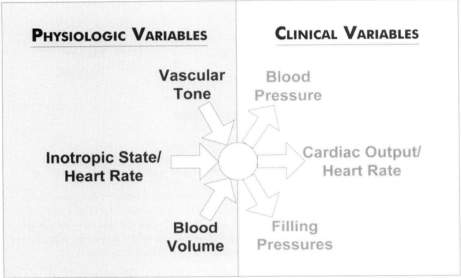

Figure 3-9. *Interrelationship of physiologic and clinical variables in heart failure.*

☑ *Physiologic changes lead to clinical changes.*

3. VENTRICULAR FUNCTION VARIABLES
(CONTRACTILITY, AFTERLOAD, PRELOAD, HEART RATE)

Ventricular function variables (or determinants) are derived from a model of the function of the heart as a pump and are estimated from clinical variables. Determinants of ventricular function include *Preload, Afterload, Contractility and Heart Rate.* Whereas, inotropic state as a physiologic variable implies myocardial force of contraction at the cellular level, contractility as a ventricular function variable includes the regional variations of timing and force of contraction across the ventricle. For example, nonuniformity in ventricular contraction or relaxation could affect the efficiency of ventricular pressure generation or ejection of blood. Both are intrinsic properties of the heart independent of afterload or preload. Heart rate is a physiologic, clinical, and ventricular function variable.

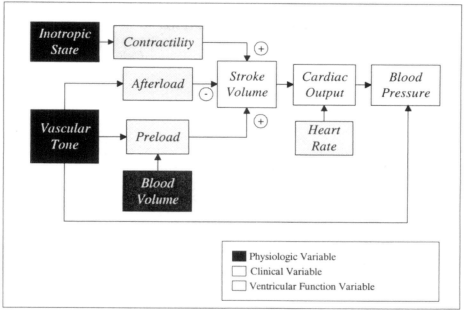

Figure 3-10. *Relationship between cardiovascular variables.*

Indices Used to Assess Ventricular Function

Selecting an index of cardiac performance depends on the desired use (see table next page). For a baseline assessment of a patient's level of systolic function or contractility, an echocardiogram can determine ejection fraction and ventricular size.

DETECTION OF ACUTE CHANGES IN CONTRACTILITY

To detect acute changes in contractility in a research cardiac catheterization laboratory, LV Peak +dP/dt or end-systolic ventricular pressure versus volume relationships can be measured (see pages 54, 57).

☑ *Ejection fraction is the best clinical index to determine baseline ventricular systolic function.*

Determinant	Measurable Indices

Contractility	Ejection fraction
	Maximum ventricular isovolumic systolic rate of
	    pressure rise (Peak +dP/dt)[3]
	Ratio of end-systolic ventricular pressure to
	    volume (Ees)[4]

Preload	Left ventricular end-diastolic volume (LVEDV) Left ventricular end-diastolic pressure (LVEDP) Pulmonary capillary wedge pressure Right atrial pressure
Afterload	Mean systolic blood pressure Systemic vascular resistance Left ventricular end-systolic wall stress
Heart Rate	Beats per minute

Relationship Between Filling Pressures and Blood Volume

Increases in intravascular or circulating blood volume will lead to increases in both right and left ventricular filling pressures. The patient with heart failure has a high vascular tone secondary to neurohormonal activation and chronic changes in vessel wall structure.[5] Increased vascular tone (and thus reduced venous capacitance) associated with heart failure will result in a greater increase in filling pressure for any given change in intravascular volume.

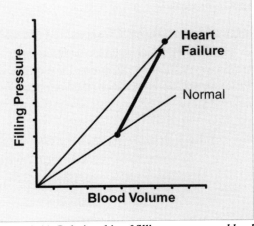

Figure 3-11. *Relationship of filling pressure vs. blood volume.*

☑ *Heart failure is associated with increases in vascular tone, blood volume, and filling pressures.*

Relationship Between Cardiac Output and Vascular Tone

Vascular tone is also a determinant of preload — via venous capacitance — and afterload — via arterial capacitance and resistance — of the right and left ventricles. Performance of the failing heart is sensitive to changes in vascular tone. Reducing vascular tone with a vasodilator drug (for example, nitroprusside) will generally lead to a biphasic response in cardiac output in patients with heart failure. Initially (A), decreasing systemic afterload will increase cardiac output as long as left heart filling pressure is maintained.[6] When reduced venous capacitance leads to an inadequate left heart filling pressure (B), then cardiac output will begin to fall according to the Frank-Starling curve.

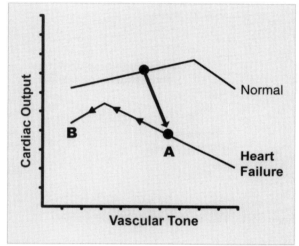

Figure 3-12. *Relationship of cardiac output vs. vascular tone.*

Interaction of the Sympathetic Nervous System and the Circulation

The sympathetic nervous system acutely adjusts circulatory function to adapt to hemodynamic perturbations, in part, through a negative feedback or closed loop system. For example, vascular pressure and stretch receptors within the carotid sinus, aorta, and cardiac chambers detect decreased blood pressure, cardiac output, or cardiac filling pressures and signal the central nervous system through afferent nerves. This results in an increase in efferent nerve traffic back to the heart and vasculature which effects a compensatory increase in blood pressure through increases in cardiac contractility and vascular smooth muscle tone.

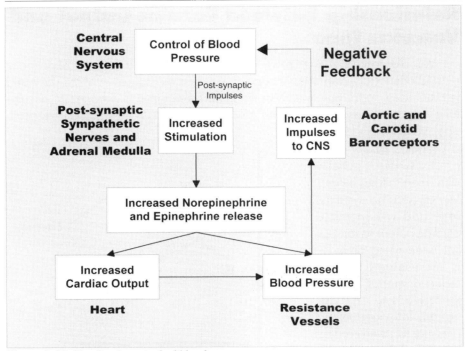

Figure 3-13. *Feedback control of blood pressure.*

   In the patient with chronic heart failure, sustained high circulating levels of catecholamines, reduced reservoirs of norepinephrine within post-synaptic sympathetic nerves, decreased intrinsic cardiac and vascular function, and down regulated sympathetic nervous system receptors all result in a loss of function of this feedback adaptive mechanism.[7-10] The circulation is functionally denervated. Loss of this control loop may contribute to circulatory instability when a hemodynamic stress challenges a patient with heart failure. Chronically, activation of the sympathetic nervous system leads to deleterious alterations in cardiac and vascular cell growth.

   ☑ *The circulation in chronic heart failure is functionally denervated.*

Orthostatic Tilt in Normal vs. Heart Failure Subjects

With a simulated stress, such as tilting patients from a supine to an upright posture, heart failure patients with normal resting hemodynamics and those with abnormal resting hemodynamics both have similar falls in pulmonary capillary wedge pressure. Heart rate increases normally in patients with normal hemodynamics, but not in more advanced patients with abnormal resting hemodynamics. This lack of responsiveness is associated with a lack of increase in plasma norepinephrine (PNE) levels in abnormal resting patients. By being in a state of high sympathetic stimulation at rest, the patient with heart failure cannot respond to acute changes in hemodynamic conditions. This sympathetic unresponsiveness may contribute to hemodynamic instability in patients with heart failure and abnormal resting hemodynamics.[11]

☑ *Resting hemodynamics and sympathetic responsiveness deteriorate from normal to abnormal as the severity of heart failure progresses.*

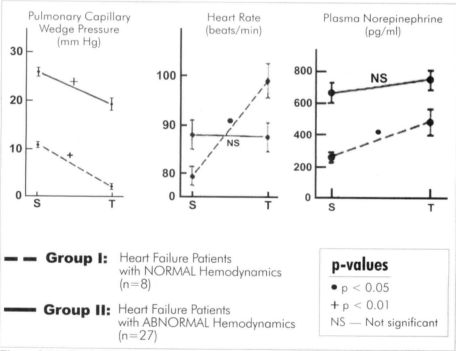

Figure 3-14. *The hemodynamic and plasma norepinephrine levels in heart failure patients with symptoms of heart failure with normal and abnormal hemodynamics during supine rest (S) and 60° orthostatic tilt (T).* Reproduced with permission. (Levine, TB et al. The neurohumoral and hemodynamic responses to orthostatic tilt in patients with congestive heart failure. Circulation 1983; 67:1071).[11]

Forearm Vascular Resistance in Normal vs. Heart Failure Subjects

Similarly, when acute intravascular volume depletion is simulated by applying a lower body negative pressure (LBNP) to patients with left ventricular dysfunction (LVD) and to controls without known heart disease (normals), vascular resistance increases in normals, consistent with vascular receptor mediated reflex vasoconstriction. No change in elevated control forearm vascular resistance occurs in patients with heart failure. Thus, the patient with advanced heart failure progressively becomes unable to compensate from either a cardiac or vascular standpoint to hemodynamic stress.[12]

☑ *Patients with end-stage heart failure are unable to adjust to acute changes in hemodynamics.*

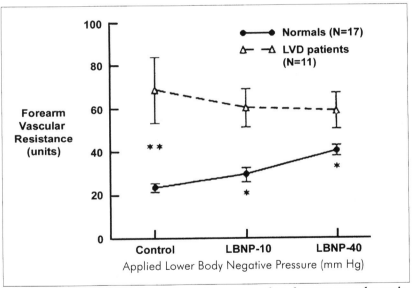

Figure 3-15. *Responses of hemodynamics measured as forearm vascular resistance in normal individuals and heart failure patients when lower body negative pressure (LBNP) is applied.* Reproduced with permission. (Ferguson et al. Selective impairment of baroreflex-mediated vasoconstrictor responses in patients with ventricular dysfunction. Circulation 1984; 69:454).[12]

Plasma Norepinephrine Predicts Prognosis

Neurohormonal activation implies a poor prognosis for the patient with heart failure. The circulating level of the primary sympathetic nervous system neurotransmitter, norepinephrine, was the most significant single predictor of survival in 642 patients in the VA Heart Failure Trial (V-HeFT I).[7]

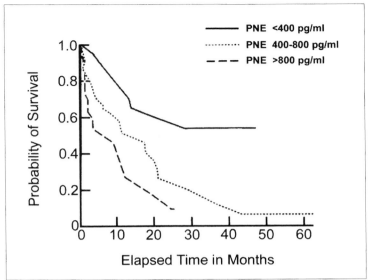

Figure 3-16. *Levels of plasma norepinephrine (PNE) related to probability of survival in V-HeFT I (VA Heart Failure Trial).* Reprinted with permission from The New England Journal of Medicine, copyright © 1984 Massachusetts Medical Society. All rights reserved. (New England Journal of Medicine, 1984; 311:822).[7]

NEUROHORMONAL ACTIVATION

Beyond identifying patients who have more advanced heart failure, neurohormonal activation may promote the progression of heart failure. Individuals with catecholamine producing tumors (pheochromocytoma) can develop dilated cardiomyopathy that returns to normal when the tumor is removed.[13] The finding that reducing adrenergic stimulation with the oral α and β adrenergic receptor blocker, carvedilol, improves survival in patients with heart failure supports this conclusion (see pages 175-177). Proof that the mechanism of benefit is secondary to direct myocardial effects beyond those due to changes in loading conditions alone requires extrapolation from animal data.

Interaction of the Renin-Angiotensin-Aldosterone System (RAAS) and the Circulation

Similar to the sympathetic nervous system, the renin-angiotensin-aldosterone system functions as a negative feedback loop. Acutely, angiotensin II acts as a potent vasoconstrictor. It also stimulates release of aldosterone at the adrenal gland cortex and antidiuretic vasopressin from the posterior pituitary gland that contribute to increases of blood volume through its effects on the kidney to promote salt and free water reabsorption.[14]

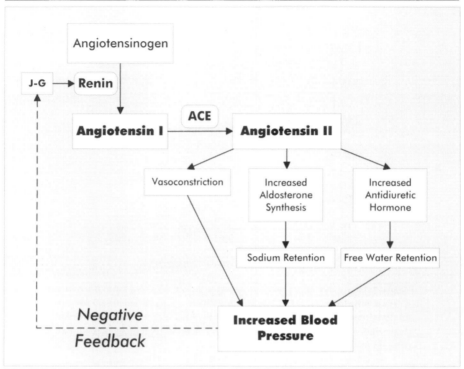

Figure 3-17. *Basic pathway of the Renin-Angiotensin-Aldosterone System (RAAS).*

KIDNEY AND ANGIOTENSIN

Juxtaglomerular (J-G) cells of the kidney release the proteolytic enzyme renin in response to a decrease in blood pressure or renal perfusion generating angiotensin I from circulating angiotensinogen. Angiotensin converting enzyme (ACE) cleavage of angiotensin II from angiotensin I in the lung produces circulating angiotensin II. However, angiotensin II can also be *formed* and *act* locally within the heart or arterial vasculature.[15] Similarly, preliminary findings suggest that aldosterone may be synthesized locally within the heart.[16]

ADDITIONAL EFFECTS OF ALDOSTERONE

In addition to effects on the kidney to enhance sodium reabsorption, aldosterone receptors are also present on cardiac fibroblasts and mediate increases in myocardial fibrosis.[16,17] Aldosterone can also contribute to the depressed responsiveness of carotid baroreceptor activity known to be present in heart failure.[17,18]

These effects may be clinically relevant. First, aldosterone levels correlated with mortality in a multicenter study of patients with advanced heart failure.[19] Second, giving an aldosterone antagonist, spironolactone, improved survival in patients with chronic heart failure.[20]

ACE INHIBITORS

ACE inhibitors are useful in chronic heart failure by multiple mechanisms.[21-23] They are potent vasodilators through at least five mechanisms: decreased angiotensin II and norepinephrine; increased bradykinin, nitric oxide, and prostaglandins.[24] By reducing the release of the hormones aldosterone and antidiuretic hormone, they reduce salt and water retention. They reduce sympathetic nerve release of norepinephrine by acting on receptors at the sympathetic nerve terminal. Finally, they reduce the effects of angiotensin as a myocardial cell growth factor (see page 89).

☑ *ACE inhibitors have beneficial effects beyond those of pure vasodilators.*

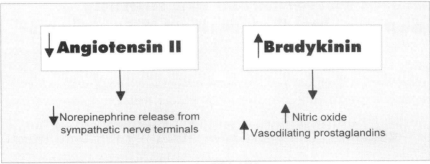

Figure 3-18. *Neurohormonal effects of ACE inhibitors.*

Mortality Increases with Chronic Use of Positive Inotropes

THE NEUROHORMONAL HYPOTHESIS

Beyond hemodynamic effects alone, endogenous or exogenous neurohormonal stimulation of the cardiovascular system in chronic heart failure leads to progressive circulatory dysfunction and subsequent increased morbidity and mortality.[25]

Acutely, neurohormonal activation or inotropic drug therapy can improve hemodynamics, but chronically can lead to adverse consequences of increased morbidity and mortality. In clinical trials, long-term administration of drugs that increase contractility in patients with heart failure has led to an increase in mortality compared to placebo.[26]

☑ *Whipping the heart leads it to burn brightly, but briefly.*

Positive Inotropic Drug	Increase in Mortality Compared to Placebo
48-hour infusions of dobutamine weekly[27]	136%
Oral flosequinan (PROFILE)[28]	51%
Oral milrinone (PROMISE)[26]	28 %

Figure 3-19. *Effects of positive inotropic drugs on mortality.*[26-28]

Neurohormonal Responses to Impaired Cardiac Performance are Initially Adaptive, but Deleterious if Sustained

In healthy individuals, circulation regulatory mechanisms respond appropriately to acute reductions in circulating blood volume. These responses lead to short-term compensatory effects. In the patient with cardiac dysfunction, however, long-term effects are often deleterious and are, therefore, targets of therapy.[29]

Response	Short-term Effects	Long-term Effects
Salt and water retention	Augments preload	Pulmonary congestion, Anasarca
Vasoconstriction	Maintains blood pressure for perfusion of vital organs (brain, heart)	Exacerbates pump dysfunction (excessive afterload), increases cardiac energy expenditure
Sympathetic stimulation	Increases heart rate and ejection	Increases energy expenditure

Figure 3-20. *Neurohormonal effects of impaired cardiac performance and their effects on the circulation.*[29]

☑ *Reflex neurohormonal action may have evolved to compensate for decreased cardiac output and blood pressure associated with acute blood loss.*

Effects of Neurohormones and Cytokine Stimulation on the Heart and the Systemic Vasculature in Heart Failure

Following a primary myocardial injury, such as acute myocardial infarction or viral myocarditis, the onset of symptoms of pump failure may occur immediately, follow days of fluid retention, or follow years of maladaptive ventricular remodeling.

Paradoxically in heart failure, peripheral responses to decreased ventricular function can contribute to symptoms of congestion and inadequate tissue perfusion. Increased levels of neurohormone mediators acting as growth factors can also promote the progression of adverse ventricular dilatation.

Not all growth factors are deleterious. In a preliminary study, administration of human growth hormone to patients with heart failure led to long-term benefits in left ventricular function.[30]

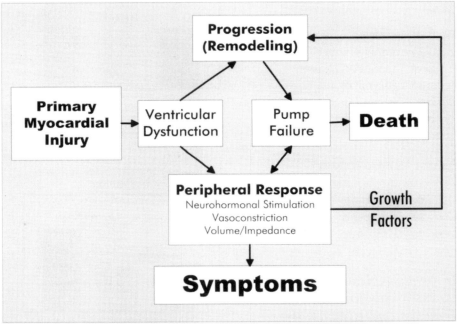

Figure 3-21. *Effects of neurohormones and cytokine stimulation on the heart and the systemic vasculature in heart failure.* Figure adapted with permission from Adis International Inc. (Cohn, JN. Vasodilators in heart failure. Conclusions from V-HeFT II and rationale for V-HeFT III. Drugs 1994; 47 Suppl 4:53).[31]

Activation of Neurohormonal Systems in Patients with Heart Failure

The patient with heart failure can manifest a progressive increase in virtually all neurohormonal systems with cardiovascular actions. Long-term effects of these systems on myocardial and vascular cell gene expression and protein translation can be important chronically.[32]

SOLVD Trials

The Studies of Left Ventricular Dysfunction (SOLVD) trials evaluated baseline levels of circulating neurohormones in three groups of individuals: normal subjects without heart disease (Control group), patients with a left ventricular ejection fraction less than 0.35 prior to the development of heart failure symptoms (Prevention group), and patients with recent development of heart failure symptoms (Treatment group).

Norepinephrine

Concordant with the V-HeFT I findings, the SOLVD levels of plasma norepinephrine corresponded to the clinical severity of heart impairment among these three groups.

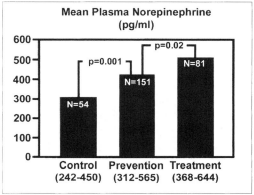

Figure 3-22. *Plasma norepinephrine in SOLVD patient groups.*

Plasma Renin Activity

Plasma renin activity, an indicator of angiotensin II formation, also increased within the three SOLVD groups.

☑ *Decreased cardiac output and low blood pressure due to heart failure may activate reflex neurohormonal changes.*

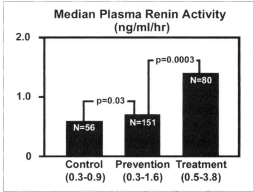

Figure 3-23. *Plasma renin activity in SOLVD patient groups.* Figures 3-22 and 3-23 reproduced with permission. (Francis GS, et al. Comparison of neuroendocrine activation in patients with left ventricular dysfunction with and without congestive heart failure. A substudy of the Studies of Left Ventricular Dysfunction (SOLVD). Circulation 1990; 82:1727).[32]

VASOPRESSIN/ANTIDIURETIC HORMONE

The posterior pituitary gland releases the vasoconstrictor and antidiuretic vasopressin, also called antidiuretic hormone, in response to systemic hypoperfusion detected via cardiac and vascular stretch receptors. Angiotensin II also stimulates vasopressin release.

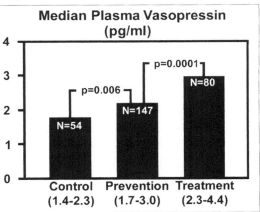

Figure 3-24. *Levels of vasopressin/antidiuretic hormones in the SOLVD patient groups.*

ATRIAL NATRIURETIC FACTOR

Normally, atrial natriuretic factor (ANF) or peptide (ANP) release from the right and left atria increases with increased atrial pressure and stretch. In chronic heart failure, patients have elevated levels of ANF to compensate for volume and pressure overload. Additionally, ventricular myocytes — which do not normally express ANF after fetal life — may adapt by synthesizing ANF. In the short-term, an increase in ANF can be beneficial by causing vasodilation and sodium and water excretion. Ultimately, however, the salutary effects of ANF are offset by tachyphylaxis and the effects of other neurohormonal mediators.[33]

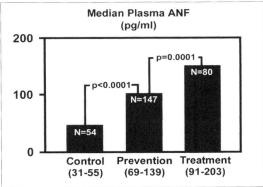

Figure 3-25. *Levels of atrial natriuretic hormone in the SOLVD patient groups.* Figures 3-24 and 3-25 reproduced with permission. (Francis GS, et al. Comparison of neuroendocrine activation in patients with left ventricular dysfunction with and without congestive heart failure. A substudy of the Studies of Left Ventricular Dysfunction (SOLVD). Circulation 1990; 82:1727).[32]

Other Mediators Involved in the Progression of Heart Failure

Besides the catecholamine and renin-angiotensin-aldosterone systems, an increasing number of additional mediators have been identified as important short-term vasoactive agents and long-term growth factors. With the exception of nitric oxide (a single nitrogen atom bonded to a single oxygen atom) and the prostaglandins, all are polypeptide molecules.[2] Refer to Figure 3-26 for these mediators and their impact on heart failure.

	EXAMPLE	SOURCE	STIMULI FOR RELEASE	EFFECTS
VASOPRESSIN	Anti-diuretic Hormone	Posterior pituitary	Hypo-perfusion Angiotensin II Hyperosmolarity Inhibited by atrial stretch	Vasoconstriction Increased free water reabsorption at distal tubule
NATRIURETIC PEPTIDES	ANP (ANF) BNP CNP	Atrium > Ventricle Ventricle > Atrium Vasculature	Increased atrial and ventricular filling pressures	Vasodilation Natriuresis Increased free water clearance
ENDOTHELIN	Endothelin - 1 Endothelin - 2 Endothelin - 3	Vascular endothelium Myocytes	Endothelin Norepinephrine Angiotensin II Thrombin TGF-β IL-1	Vasoconstriction Myocardial fibrosis

Figure 3-26. *Mediators involved in the progression of heart failure.*[2]

	EXAMPLE	SOURCE	STIMULI FOR RELEASE	EFFECTS
NITRIC OXIDE	Endothelium derived relaxing factor (EDRF)	Vascular endothelium Myocytes	Acetylcholine Thrombin Other mediators Blood flow Shear stress	Vasodilation Negative inotrope
CYTOKINES	TNF-α Interleukin I Interferons	Monocytes Lymphocytes Fibroblasts Myocytes	Hemodynamic overload Norepinephrine Other cytokines	Modulate gene expression Negative inotrope
KININS	Bradykinin	Cleaved from plasma kinogen by vascular kallikrein (esp. renal)	Low sodium intake Aldosterone	Vasodilation Increased EDRF, PGE_2, PGI_2
PROSTAGLANDINS Vasodilators	PGE_2, PGI_2 (prostacyclin)	Vascular endothelium and smooth muscle (esp. renal)	Decreased renal blood flow Vasoconstrictors HDL	Vasodilation
Vasoconstrictors	Thromboxane	Platelet	Platelet activation	Vasoconstriction

William Harvey
(1578-1657)

Prior to the time of William Harvey, physicians believed that blood in the veins and arteries oscillated to and from the heart to heat the blood and provide vital substances to the body. Blood "created" in the liver was thought to reach the left ventricle by passing from the right ventricle through "invisible pores" in the ventricular septum. Harvey discovered the circulation of the blood and helped initiate the application of experimental methods to medicine.[34]

Harvey, a native of England, was 22 years old when he traveled to the University of Padua in Italy to study medicine. He thought about the abundance and orientation of venous valves directing blood toward the heart, including those in neck veins that would have nothing to do with gravity. He, like others, noted that venous valves resembled heart valves in structure. Subsequently, he did experiments to show quantitatively that the amount of blood pumped by the heart would quickly exhaust the entire blood volume if it did not return in a circular fashion back to the heart. Although Harvey did not have a microscope to see the capillaries that connected the body's arteries to the veins, he postulated that they had to exist.

Harvey was the first to accurately describe blood circulation based on his gradual collection of diverse anatomic and functional observations about blood vessels and the heart.

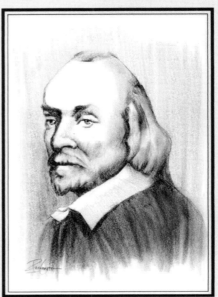

Figure 3-27. *William Harvey. Illustration by Peter Chapman.*

Chapter 3 Quiz

1. A patient has high filling pressures, depressed cardiac index, and normal blood pressure. The patient most likely has which type of heart failure?
    a) new onset heart failure
    b) decompensated heart failure
    c) compensated heart failure
    d) none of the above

2. Check (√) the value(s) below that are consistent with decompensated heart failure hemodynamics:

    _____ CO = 2.5 L/min   _____ PCW = 30 mm Hg
    _____ HR = 120 bpm   _____ SVR = 1500 dyne sec cm^{-5}
    _____ RA = 4 mm Hg   _____ EF = 20%

3. Patients with heart failure may have depressed oxygen consumption during exercise due to which of the following?
    a) decreased stroke volume
    b) decreased blood pressure
    c) decreased respiratory rate

4. Each of the following is a phase of the cardiac cycle except:
    a) isovolumic diastole
    b) systolic ejection
    c) isovolumic relaxation
    d) diastolic filling

5. An increase in vascular tone will lead to all of the following except:
    a) increased venous capacitance
    b) increased LV afterload
    c) increased arterial pulse pressure
    d) decreased systemic vascular resistance

6. Drugs may improve myocardial ischemia in failing hearts by:
    a) increasing contractility to reduce myocardial oxygen consumption
    b) decreasing contractility to increase myocardial oxygen consumption
    c) decreasing afterload to increase myocardial oxygen consumption
    d) decreasing afterload to reduce myocardial oxygen consumption

7. The following are considered to be measurable "clinical" variables associated with heart failure except:
    a) blood pressure
    b) vascular tone
    c) filling pressures
    d) cardiac output

8. Which of the following is not a measurable index of ventricular preload?
    a) pulmonary capillary wedge pressure
    b) systemic vascular resistance
    c) left ventricular end-diastolic volume
    d) left ventricular end-diastolic pressure

9. Patients with heart failure typically have high vascular tone secondary to neurohormonal activation and chronic changes in vessel wall structure. This increase in vascular tone can result in which of the following?
    a) a greater increase in filling pressure with decreased blood volume
    b) a lower increase in filling pressure with increased blood volume
    c) a greater increase in filling pressure with increased blood volume
    d) a greater decrease in filling pressure with increased blood volume

10. All of the following contribute to the loss of control of the negative feedback loop in the neurohormonal activation of heart failure except:
    a) sustained high circulating levels of catecholamines
    b) increased reservoirs of norepinephrine within post-synaptic
        sympathetic nerves
    c) decreased intrinsic cardiac and vascular function
    d) down regulation of sympathetic nervous system receptors

11. Long-term inotropic drug therapy can improve both quality of life and potential for long-term survival through significant increases in hemody-namic function in patients with heart failure.
    a) true
    b) false

12. Chronic effects of reflex neurohormonal action (i.e., salt and water retention, vasoconstriction, and sympathetic stimulation) include:
    a) pulmonary congestion
    b) increased cardiac energy expenditure
    c) anasarca
    d) all of the above

13. The SOLVD trial showed that all of the following circulating neurohormones were associated with the progression of heart failure except:
    a) norepinephrine
    b) nitric oxide
    c) arginine vasopressin
    d) atrial natriuretic factor

See Appendix for solutions.

Organ

Chapter 4

This chapter describes functional and structural changes that accompany systolic and diastolic heart failure. An understanding of these alterations provides the basis for therapy of patient symptoms and long-term disease management.

The Heart as a Target Organ

Heart failure is the potential end-result of any process that adversely affects heart function. A diagnosis of heart failure should attempt to include specific etiologies whenever possible.

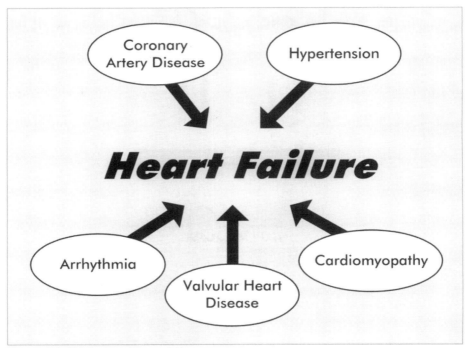

Figure 4-1. *Etiologies of heart failure.*

☑ *Heart failure is the end result of any process that adversely affects cardiac function.*

Electrical and Pressure Events in Systole and Diastole

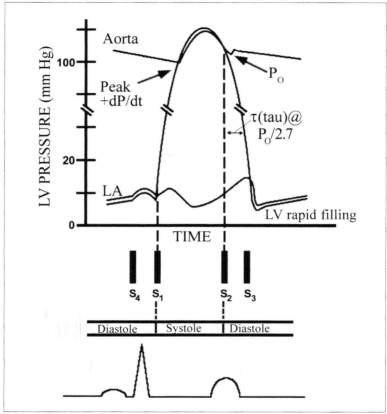

Figure 4-2. *Electrical and pressure events in systole and diastole. τ (tau) — the exponential time constant describing pressure decrease within the left ventricle following aortic valve closure, an index of diastolic function. Peak +dP/dt — peak rate of left ventricular pressure increase during isovolumic systole, an index of systolic function.*

Electrical events control the mechanical actions of systole and diastole. A clinical definition of left ventricular (LV) systole is the interval between mitral valve closure and aortic valve closure. The mitral valve closes when LV pressure exceeds left atrial (LA) pressure after electrical ventricular activation. Similarly, the aortic valve closes when ventricular relaxation results in LV pressure falling below aortic pressure. Heart sounds occur with these two valve closure events: S_1 and S_2 respectively. In patients with heart failure, additional heart sounds can be audible occurring with LV rapid filling, S_3, or left atrial contraction, S_4.

Circulatory Flow Patterns

The right and left ventricles are pumps that take the circulation of blood from low venous to high arterial pressure vascular reservoirs. Continuous venous return phasically enters the atria. Biphasic flow crosses the AV valves only during diastole aided by ventricular suction and atrial contraction. Flow across the aortic and pulmonary valves is a single pulsatile systolic bolus. The net flow into versus out of atrial and ventricular chambers determines their instantaneous volumes. Total heart volume (myocardial solid plus chamber blood volumes) remains approximately the same at end-diastole and end-systole with balanced changes in atrial and ventricular volume during alternate phases of the cardiac cycle.[1]

☑ *Echocardiography with Doppler allows assessment of chamber volumes and flows.*

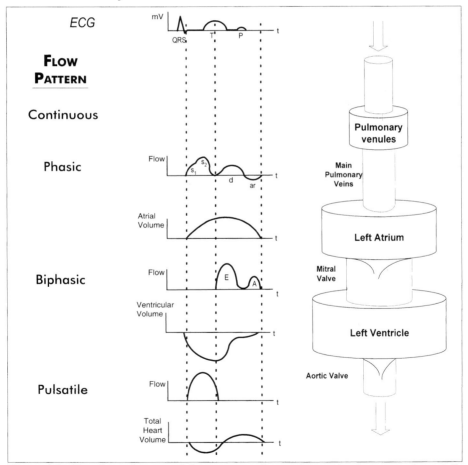

Figure 4-3. Chamber volumes and flows. s_1, s_2— *first and second pulmonary vein systolic flow, respectively; d — pulmonary vein diastolic flow; ar — atrial reversal flow; E— early filling; A — atrial contraction.*

Ventricular Pressure-Volume Relationships

Plotting the cardiac cycle as a pressure-volume work performing pump with ventricular pressure on the vertical axis and ventricular volume on the horizontal axis can provide a model of heart failure secondary to either systolic or diastolic dysfunction. The area of the pressure-volume loop represents work.

THE HEART AS A WORK PERFORMING MECHANICAL PUMP

As a mechanical pump, the heart operates within the limits imposed by the end-systolic and diastolic ventricular pressure-volume relationships (Figure 4-4). The smaller the spread between these two operating curves, the more severe the impairment in the function of the heart as a pump. From the perspective of the heart as a pressure-volume pump, a goal of therapy should be to increase the spread between the end-systolic and diastolic relations.

SYSTOLIC AND DIASTOLIC DYSFUNCTION

Systolic dysfunction occurs when the end-systolic pressure-volume curve moves downward or to the right. Diastolic dysfunction occurs when the diastolic curve moves upward or to the left. In the extreme, no pump action would be possible if the systolic and diastolic curves overlapped.

☑ *From the perspective of the heart as a pressure-volume pump, a goal of therapy should be to increase the spread between the end-systolic and diastolic relations.*

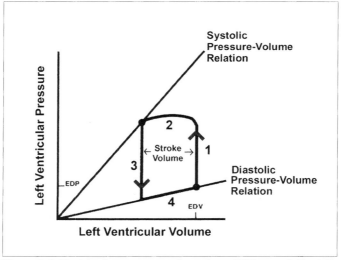

Figure 4-4. *Ventricular pressure-volume loop. EDP — end-diastolic pressure; EDV — end-diastolic volume.*

Systolic Dysfunction

When ventricular *systolic* dysfunction occurs, the end-systolic pressure-volume curve moves from 1 to 2. This can lead to a decrease in systolic pressure, stroke volume, and ejection fraction despite a compensatory increase in the operating point on the dias-tolic pressure-volume curve.

☑ *Contractility can be defined by the slope of the end-systolic pres-sure-volume curve.*

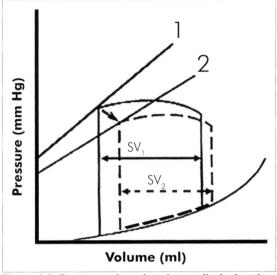

Figure 4-5. *Pressure-volume loop in systolic dysfunction.*

Diastolic Dysfunction

When ventricular *diastolic* dysfunction occurs, the dias-tolic pressure-volume curve shifts from 1 to 2. This can lead to an increase in dias-tolic pressure, a decrease in end-diastolic volume, and a decrease in ventricular stroke volume. Diastolic dysfunction can occur with or without as-sociated systolic dysfunction. For example, a patient with hypertensive heart disease can have diastolic dysfunction resulting in pulmonary edema with a normal or increased ejection fraction.

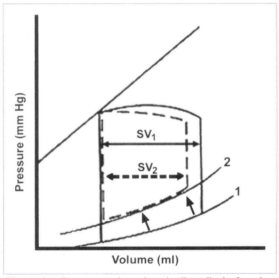

Figure 4-6. *Pressure-volume loop in diastolic dysfunction.*

☑ *Diastolic function can be defined by the diastolic pressure-volume relationship.*

Systolic and Diastolic Dysfunction and the Frank-Starling Curve

A decrease in a Frank-Starling left ventricular performance curve typically implies a decrease in systolic function. A decrease in diastolic ventricular chamber compliance, however, will also result in a downward shift of this curve when left ventricular filling pressure is the horizontal axis variable. With diastolic dysfunction, the left ventricle requires a higher end-diastolic pressure to achieve the same end-diastolic volume and stretch of actin and myosin filaments to subsequently eject the same stroke volume. Thus, although a Frank-Starling curve can depict left ventricular performance over a range of preloads, one cannot distinguish a systolic *versus* diastolic mechanism of a change in performance (for example, from a to b) from this model alone.

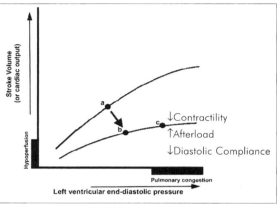

Figure 4-7. *The Frank-Starling curve demonstrates left ventricluar performance, but does not differentiate between systolic and diastolic dysfunction.*

USE OF DIASTOLIC VOLUME AND PRESSURE

When using the Frank-Starling curve and pressure-volume loop models together in a given clinical situation, you should recognize that ventricular diastolic *volume* determines ventricular preload for systolic performance, but diastolic *pressure* determines the potential for end-organ congestion such as pulmonary edema.

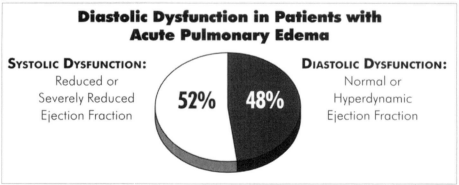

Figure 4-8. *Of the patients presenting with pulmonary edema, approximately half had preserved left ventricular performance as measured by echocardiography and radionuclide ventriculography.*[3]

Left ventricular systolic dysfunction is the most common finding in patients with heart failure. As many as half of patients presenting with *acute pulmonary edema*, however, have preserved systolic function by echocardiography, particularly in the elderly. In the absence of significant valvular or pericardial disease, these patients have diastolic dysfunction. Diastolic dysfunction is associated with hypertension, increasing age, diabetes mellitus, and female gender.[2] Typically, the left ventricular internal chamber dimension is normal by echocardiography even if cardiomegaly is present on chest x-ray due to increased left ventricular wall thickness or atrial chamber size. In a study by Bier and colleagues, 42 of 87 patients with acute pulmonary edema had a preservation of ejection fraction by echocardiography and radionuclide ventriculography.[3]

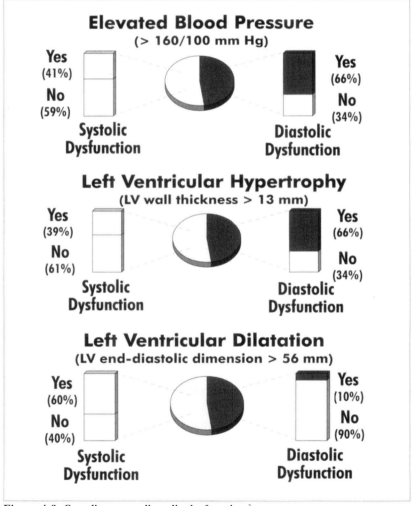

Figure 4-9. *Systolic versus diastolic dysfunction.*[3]

Wall Stress within the Myocardium: LaPlace's Law

Wall stress, σ, is the local force acting on myocytes within the left ventricle that determines their load (see page 274). This load is important because it determines regional myocyte performance and energy consumption.[4]

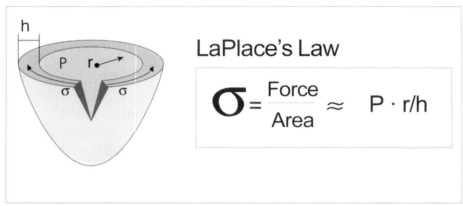

Figure 4-10. *LaPlace's Law as it relates to myocardial wall stress. P — pressure; r — chamber radius; h — wall thickness; σ — wall stress.*

MEASURING WALL STRESS

One can measure wall stress in contracting *in vitro* preparations of heart papillary muscle, but not in the intact contracting heart. Estimates of *in vivo* wall stress, however, are possible using a geometric model of the heart as a thick-walled rotated ellipse. Exact solutions of this depend on the location and direction of force generated with the ventricular wall.

LaPLACE'S LAW APPLIED TO THE HEART

La Place's Law ($σ = P \cdot r/h$) can have major implications for an injured heart that dilates to permit an increase in an inadequate stroke volume. A dilated heart (increased r) maintains a systolic pressure at the cost of a higher systolic wall stress load on myocytes. Conversely, a dilated heart has a blunted maximum ventricular pressure generation with myocytes that contract with only a limited force (or wall stress). Developing a thicker wall (increased h) can offset this, but at the potential of increased chamber stiffness or myocardial ischemia.

> ☑ *Increased heart chamber diameter increases myocardial wall stress during contraction.*

CHRONIC EFFECTS OF INCREASED WALL STRESS

Chronically, increased systolic or diastolic wall stress is associated with ventricular remodeling and subsequent wall hypertrophy and chamber enlargement.

Concentric vs. Dilated Hypertrophy

The normal left ventricle surrounds a rotated ellipse or football shaped chamber with end-diastolic wall thickness less than or equal to 11 mm and chamber diameter less than or equal to 56 mm. A normal left ventricular size can also be defined based on a calculated estimate of left ventricular mass corrected for body size or surface area. During systolic wall thickening and ejection of blood, the base of the left ventricle, including the mitral and aortic valves, moves toward a relatively stationary apex.[5]

CONCENTRIC HYPERTROPHY (SMALL LEFT VENTRICLE OR CHAMBER)

Concentric hypertrophy can develop in response to a sustained increase in left ventricular systolic pressure. End-diastolic wall thickness, h, will increase and the chamber radius, r, and volume will decrease. Since by the LaPlace relation, wall stress at end-systole is reduced, ejection fraction (EF) may initially increase to maintain a constant stroke volume. A left ventricle subjected to long-standing pressure overload, however, can progress to a dilated ventricle with dilated hypertrophy.

DILATED HYPERTROPHY (ENLARGED LEFT VENTRICLE OR CHAMBER)

Dilated hypertrophy can follow myocardial injury (infarction, myocarditis) or a chronic volume overload (for example, aortic or mitral valve regurgitation). Initially, an increase in heart size achieved by passive stretch will maintain a forward stroke volume via the Frank-Starling mechanism. Remodelling further increases chamber size over time. Increased heart size ultimately decreases ventricular ejection if increased systolic wall stress and tension create an excessive afterload for contracting myocytes.

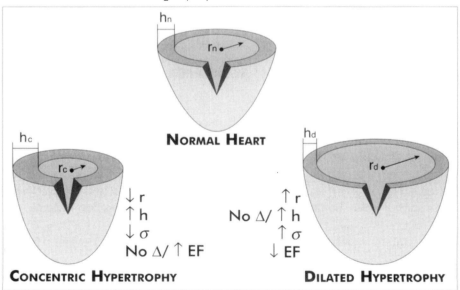

Figure 4-11. *Concentric and dilated hypertrophy. r — chamber radius; h — wall thickness; σ — wall stress; EF — ejection fraction.*

Hypothesis: Increased Wall Stress Initiates Concentric and Dilated Hypertrophy

Grossman and colleagues proposed that increased wall stress signals myocyte growth to continue until wall stress returns to normal. This hypothesis requires that the heart can "detect" systolic and diastolic wall stress occurring with pressure and volume overload, respectively. Stretch of membrane proteins or changes in intracellular calcium ion concentration within the myocyte or associated fibroblasts may permit the cell to do this. Locally synthesized angiotensin II may serve an intermediate role and act as a growth factor in a paracrine (on neighboring cells), autocrine (on the same cell), or intracrine (internally on the same cell without extracellular secretion) mode.[6]

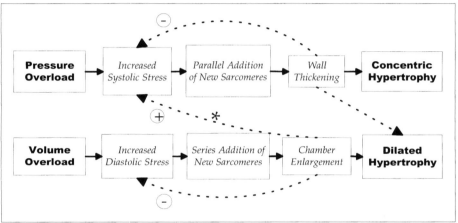

Figure 4-12. *Hypothesized mechanism by which increased wall stress initiates concentric and dilated hypertrophy.* Adapted from The Journal of Clinical Investigation, 1975; 56:61 by copyright permission of The American Society for Clinical Investigation.[7]

ADDITION OF NEW SARCOMERES

In addition, a control mechanism is necessary to selectively and appropriately add new sarcomeres in either a parallel or series position to return wall stress toward normal. How the myocyte does this is unknown. With a chronic *volume* overload (see Figure 4-12) (*), chamber enlargement ($\uparrow$ r) and the LaPlace relation ($\sigma = P \cdot r/h$) result in an increased systolic and diastolic wall stress so that both chamber enlargement *and* wall thickening can occur.

Stages of Cardiac Disease

The clinical syndrome of heart failure (circulatory congestion or inadequate tissue perfusion) may be similar regardless of the etiology of primary damage or mechanism of systolic versus diastolic dysfunction. Systolic dysfunction usually predominates following myocardial infarction, diffuse viral or idiopathic cardiomyopathy, or chronic volume overload. Diastolic dysfunction due to left ventricular concentric hypertrophy develops with systemic hypertension, aortic stenosis, or hypertrophic cardiomyopathy. Eventually, concentric hypertrophy may progress to ventricular chamber enlargement and systolic dysfunction if long-standing pressure overload or myocardial ischemia occurs.[8]

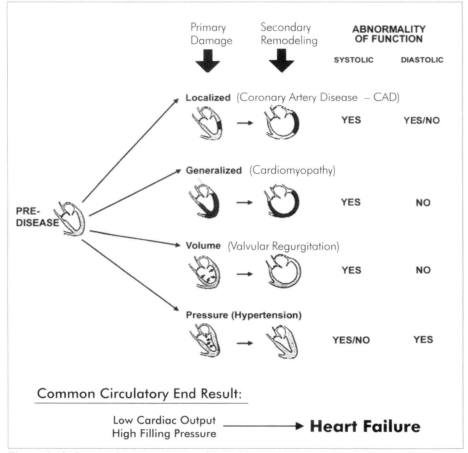

Figure 4-13. *Stages of cardiac disease. Clinical heart failure may result from various causes that produce a primary insult that proceeds to secondary remodeling.* With permission from: Gorlin R., Treatment of congestive heart failure: where are we going? Circulation 1987; 75:IV109.[8]

Pathophysiology of Diastolic Dysfunction

Decreased left ventricular relaxation, increased passive chamber stiffness, or both will lead to an upward shift in the ventricular diastolic pressure-volume curve. Patients with heart failure may have diastolic dysfunction of more than one etiology.[9]

☑ *Diastolic dysfunction may result from abnormal ventricular relaxation, passive chamber stiffness, or both.*

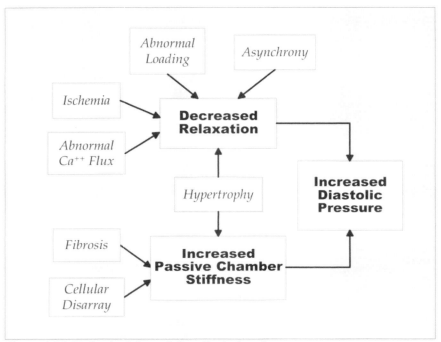

Figure 4-14. *Pathophysiology of diastolic dysfunction.*

Causes of Increased Left Ventricular Diastolic Pressure

Left ventricular diastolic dysfunction is an important cause of heart failure that may be associated with normal, reduced, or hyperdynamic systolic function. An elevated diastolic pressure within the left ventricle due to any cause can result in pulmonary congestion.

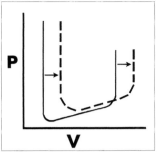

Figure 4-15. *Chamber dilation.*[6]

CHAMBER DILATION

Chamber dilation due to an increased intra-vascular volume will increase both left ventricular pressure and volume along a single diastolic pressure-volume curve. This acutely accompanies systolic dysfunction to compensate for decreased ejection of blood.

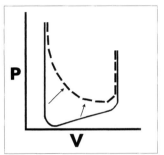

Figure 4-16. *Abnormal relaxation.*[6]

ABNORMAL RELAXATION

Ventricular relaxation is an energy requiring event affecting isovolumic relaxation, rapid ventricular filling, and mid-diastolic filling. Abnormal relaxation will result in an increase in left ventricular pressure especially in the first two-thirds of diastole.

INCREASED CHAMBER STIFFNESS

Increased chamber stiffness implies a change in the passive stretch properties of the left ventricular muscle and chamber. It will predominantly affect the last two-thirds of diastole.

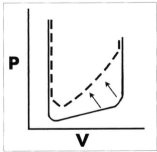

Figure 4-17. *Increased chamber stiffness.*[6]

PERICARDIAL RESTRAINT

Finally, in the absence of any change in the pressure-volume characteristics of the ventricle, changes in pericardial restraint will lead to an increase in pressure throughout diastole and a parallel shift up in the pressure vs. time or pressure vs. volume curve. It will affect the right and left ventricle equally. Even though the *transmural* pressure across the ventricle (between the ventricular chamber and the pericardial space) will be normal for any given volume, the total pressure (transmural pressure + pericardial pressure) will be increased and this pressure will reflect to the pulmonary and systemic venous circulations.

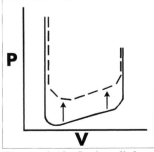

Figure 4-18. *Pericardial restraint.*[6]

Nonuniformity as a Determinant of Contraction and Relaxation

Preload, afterload, and contractility determine myocardial performance. In addition, effective contraction and relaxation require a *coordinated distribution* of ventricular *load* and *contractility*. Spatial and temporal nonuniformity of load and contractility will result in the dissipation of myocardial energy as internal work rather than pump external function and affect global ventricular performance. For example, a change in ventricular contraction induced by a left bundle branch block pattern of depolarization will lead to a loss of pump efficiency for any given end-diastolic volume, mean arterial pressure, and myocardial inotropic state.[10] In patients with heart failure and an intraventricular conduction defect, electrical pacing of either the left ventricle or simultaneous right and left ventricular chambers has been proposed as an intervention to improve ventricular function and patient outcome.[11]

☑ *Biventricular pacing may improve heart function in patients with a prolonged QRS duration.*

EFFECTS OF NONUNIFORMITY

In the absence of other impairment in ventricular function, the decrease in function with an intraventricular conduction defect would be small. With a reduced cardiac reserve in heart failure, however, the effects of nonuniformity can be substantial. Other examples include nonuniformities of contraction and relaxation due to coronary artery disease or hypertrophic cardiomyopathy.

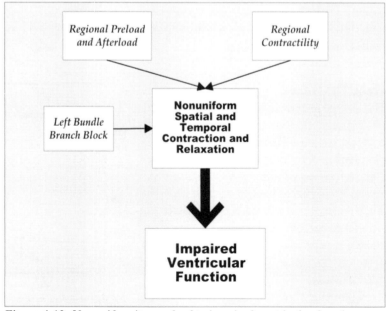

Figure 4-19. *Nonuniformity can lead to impaired ventricular function.*

Chapter 4 Quiz

1. Which of the following may contribute to the development of heart failure?
    a) coronary artery disease
    b) arrhythmia
    c) valvular heart disease
    d) hypertension
    e) all of the above

2. The total heart volume of the heart (i.e., myocardial solid plus chamber blood volumes) remains approximately the same at end-diastole and end-systole.
    a) True
    b) False

3. As a mechanical pump, the heart operates within the limits imposed by end-systolic and diastolic ventricular pressure-volume relationships. A _____ spread between the two operating curves indicates a _____ performance of the heart as a pump.
    a) larger; better
    b) smaller; better
    c) larger; similar
    d) smaller; similar

4. As compared to systolic dysfunction, diastolic dysfunction is more commonly associated with all of the following except:
    a) decreased end-diastolic volume
    b) elevated blood pressure
    c) left ventricular hypertrophy
    d) left ventricular dilatation

5. In the Frank-Starling ventricular performance curve, ventricular diastolic volume determines ventricular _____ for systolic performance and diastolic pressure determines the potential for _____.
    a) congestion; preload
    b) preload; congestion
    c) afterload; edema
    d) edema; afterload

6. Match the figure with the type of hypertrophy:
    a) normal heart
    b) concentric hypertrophy
    c) dilated hypertrophy

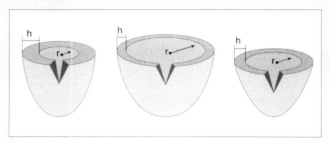

7. All of the following may contribute to decreased relaxation in diastolic dysfunction except:
    a) abnormal loading
    b) hypertrophy
    c) increased catecholamines
    d) ischemia

8. Factors which may lead to the spatial and temporal nonuniformity of load and contractility of the heart include all of the following except:
    a) left bundle branch block
    b) valvular disease
    c) coronary artery disease
    d) hypertrophic cardiomyopathy

See Appendix for solutions.

Cell

Chapter 5

This chapter examines the structure, function, and biochemical properties of cardiac and vascular cells to demonstrate potential sites for heart failure therapy.

The Cardiac Muscle Cell

Cardiac muscle is composed primarily of muscle cells, or myocytes in an extracellular matrix associated with vascular, fibrous, and blood-related cells. Intercalated discs connect myocytes to each other in a branching network forming distinct spiral bundles within the ventricle chambers. Systolic shortening of these spiral bundles leads to a twisting deformation of the ventricle with each contraction as it ejects blood.[1] Recoil of the deformed spirals contributes to early relaxation of the ventricle.

Following acute myocardial infarction, enlargement of ventricular chamber size can occur due to both early slippage of cells within their collagen matrix, and late myocyte cell lengthening within viable noninfarcted regions. Increases in the percent of left ventricular volume due to extracellular collagen may contribute to changes in left ventricular geometry. The net result is that left ventricular chamber volume increases out of proportion to left ventricular mass without change in noninfarcted left ventricular wall thickness.[2] Similar mechanisms may contribute to dilated hypertrophy in non-ischemic cardiomyopathy.[3]

MYOFIBRILS

Within each myocyte cell, repeating units of sarcomeres arranged in series form myofibrils. Myofilaments of actin and myosin are the contractile proteins that constitute each sarcomere (see Chapter 6, Sarcomere).

TRANSVERSE TUBULES (T-TUBULES)

T-tubule invaginations of the cardiac cell membrane (sarcolemma) penetrate into the myocyte to permit close contact between the high concentration of calcium in the extracellular space and the low concentration of calcium in the intracellular cytoplasm. Furthermore, the close apposition of T-tubules to intracellular calcium reservoirs within the myocyte (sarcoplasmic reticulum) allows rapid signalling for additional release of calcium and initiation of contraction.[4]

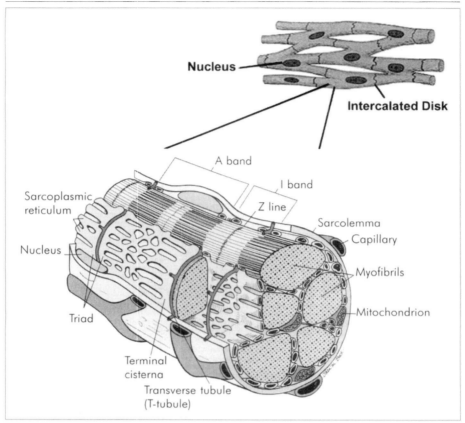

Figure 5-1. *Structure of the heart muscle.* Top from Braunwald E, Ross J, Sonnenblick E. *Mechanisms of Contraction of the Normal and Failing Heart*. Little, Brown and Company, 1976, page 3.[5] Adapted with permission from Lippincott, Williams, and Wilkins. Bottom from Schauf, Charles. *Human Physiology, Foundations and Frontiers*. Times Mirror/Mosby College Publishing, 1990, page 293. Reproduced with permission of The McGraw-Hill Companies.[6]

END-DIFFERENTIATED MYOCYTE

As an end-differentiated cell, a myocyte cannot divide but can enlarge in size with multiple nuclei in response to mechanical or biochemical stimuli. Specialized myocytes (Purkinje cells) also have electrical properties that allow the transmission of electrical stimuli to coordinate global organ contraction.

Myocyte Measurement	Description
Shape	Long and narrow
Length (μm)	60-140
Diameter (μm)	Approximately 20
Volume (μm³)	15-45,000
Intercalated disc	Prominent end-to-end connections
General appearance	Mitochondria and sarcomeres very abundant; Rectangular branching bundles with little interstitial collagen

Figure 5-2. *Description of the ventricular myocyte cell.*[7]

Myocyte Organelle	Approximate % of Cell Volume	Function
Myofibril	50-60	Interaction of thick and thin filaments during contraction cycle
Mitochondria	20-25	Provide high energy ATP chiefly for contraction and homeostasis
Nucleus	About 5	mRNA synthesis
Sarcoplasmic Reticulum (SR)	2	Takes up and releases calcium during contraction cycle
T-tubules	About 1	Transmission of electrical signal from sarcolemma to cell interior
Sarcolemma (cell membrane)	Very Low	Control of ionic gradients; channels for ions (action potential); maintenance of cell integrity; receptors for drugs and hormones
Lysosomes	Very Low	Intracellular digestion and proteolysis
Sarcoplasm (cytoplasm)	20	Provides cytosol in which rise and fall of ionized calcium occurs; contains other ions, small molecules, and proteins

Figure 5-3. *Composition of the ventricular myocyte in the adult male.*[7]

☑ *Contracting myofibrils account for about half of the myocyte cell volume.*

Oxidative Phosphorylation

The heart functions as a circulatory pump by conversion of biochemical energy to pressure-volume work through oxidative phosphorylation and utilization of adenosine triphosphate by actin and myosin. Coronary artery disease can cause acute or chronic inadequate delivery of oxygen to the heart and initiate a downhill spiral of ventricular dysfunction, systemic hypoperfusion, and death.

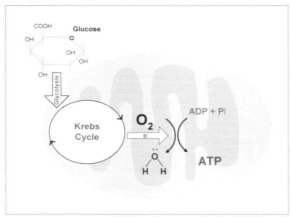

Figure 5-4. *Oxidative phosphorylation pathway.*

Energy Utilization in Heart Failure

Energy utilization per gram of heart tissue of the dilated failing heart is greater than the normal heart because of the LaPlace relationship where myocardial systolic wall tension is proportional to left ventricular chamber radius.[8] Thus, heart dilation results in greater systolic wall tension and increased myocardial oxygen consumption.

ENERGY UTILIZATION IN VENTRICULAR HYPERTROPHY

Ventricular hypertrophy can lead up to a threefold increase in left ventricular mass.[9] Maximum oxygen supply does not increase proportionately with heart hypertrophy and resting energy utilization, thus limiting energy reserve.[10]

Ventricular chamber size (and radius) can be reduced with diuretics. Surgical removal of an akinetic or dyskinetic ventricular aneurysm can also reduce ventricular radius and energy needs. Finally, Batista has proposed an experimental therapy of ventricular resection of myocardial tissue in some patients with dilated cardiomyopathy to reduce heart size and improve myocardial efficiency.[11]

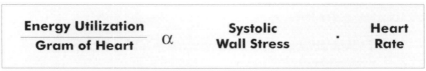

Figure 5-5. *Energy utilization in heart failure.*

Myocyte Time-course of Excitation, Calcium Release, and Contraction

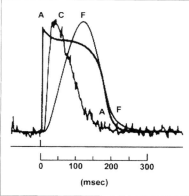

In vitro preparations of heart papillary muscle demonstrate the linked relationships between electrical depolarization, calcium ion concentration, and myocardial force generation within individual myocytes. The intervals between electrical action potential depolarization (A) to calcium release (C) and calcium release to force production (F) constitute the myocyte electromechanical interval.

$$\boxed{\checkmark}\ Depolarization \rightarrow \frac{Calcium}{Release} \rightarrow Force$$

Figure 5-6. *Myocyte excitation, calcium release, and contraction. (A) electrical action potential, (C) Ca^{++} concentration, (F) force generation.* From Braunwald, E: Heart Disease, A Textbook of Cardiovascular Medicine, 4th edition. Saunders, 1992, p. 357. In Langer, GA [ed.]: Calcium and the Heart, New York, Raven Press, 1990, p. 312. Permission granted by the copyright holder: Lippincott, Williams and Wilkins.

Myocyte Intracellular Calcium Release and Reuptake

Myocyte inotropic state depends on the delivery and reuptake of calcium to the actin component of the myofilament contractile machinery. The intracellular sarcoplasmic reticulum reservoir maintains a high calcium ion concentration similar to the extracellular space. Along with calcium entry through the cell membrane, the sarcoplasmic reticulum releases stores of calcium when the myocyte is electrically depolarized, thereby increasing intracellular concentration from a resting value of about 0.01 mmol/L to 1-10 mmol/L.[7]

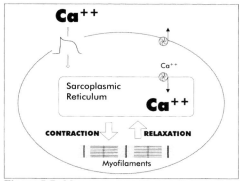

Figure 5-7. *Myocyte contraction and relaxation. Normal serum ionized calcium concentration is 1.14-1.30 mmol/L.*

MYOFILAMENT RELAXATION

ATP energy requiring calcium ion pumps in the sarcoplasmic reticulum and cell membranes effect myofilament relaxation. These protein pumps restore the high gradient for calcium between the myocyte cytoplasm and the surrounding sarcoplasmic reticulum and extracellular compartments following cell repolarization. With each heart beat, changes in calcium concentration within the myocyte determine myofilament force of contraction and rate of relaxation.

Relationship between Intracellular Calcium Concentration and Force of Contraction

Successively increasing the concentration of a positive inotrope catecholamine (isoproterenol) can yield a range of conditions of contractility in *in vitro* preparations of cardiac muscle cells. Force generation (F) per contraction is related to the increase in calcium concentration per beat (C).[12]

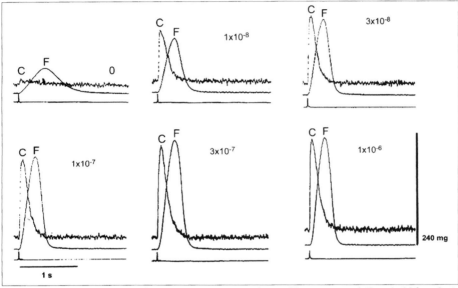

Figure 5-8. *The influence of increasing concentrations of isoproterenol (0 to 1x10⁻⁶ molar).*
Reprinted with permission from the American College of Cardiology (**Journal of the American College of Cardiology**, February 1984; 3:412).[12]

$$[Ca^{++}](time) \longrightarrow Force(time)$$

Catecholamine Receptor Types

Norepinephrine is the catecholamine molecule released by stimulated sympathetic nerve terminals. Norepinephrine effects result from the sum of activation of catecholamine receptors that vary in type and distribution by anatomic location and cell type.

β_1-receptors are the major catecholamine receptor on myocytes; activation results in an increase in cardiac contractility. Smaller numbers of β_2-receptors are also present on myocytes but these increase in proportion to β_1-receptors in patients with heart failure.[13]

α_1 catecholamine receptors predominate on vascular smooth muscle cells; activation results in vasoconstriction. β_2-receptors in skeletal muscle and dopamine receptors in renal and other abdominal organs are also present in vascular smooth muscle cells; activation results in vasodilation.

Drug therapy tailored to promote or blunt catecholamine receptor pathways underlies treatment of both acute and chronic heart failure.

EFFECTS OF CATECHOLAMINE STIMULATION

Catecholamine stimulation of the β-receptors on myocytes leads to phosphorylation of the calcium channel in the cell membrane by a c-AMP dependent protein. The phosphorylated calcium channel has a higher permeability to calcium and thus calcium accumulates intracellularly. In addition, phospholamban, a regulatory protein associated with the sarcoplasmic reticulum calcium pump, becomes phosphorylated (see page 97). This increases the rate of calcium reuptake by the sarcoplasmic reticulum and subsequent delivery of calcium with cell depolarization. Thus, both myocardial relaxation and force of contraction increase.

HEART FAILURE AND REDUCED RESPONSE TO CATECHOLAMINES

Papillary muscles from patients with end-stage idiopathic cardiomyopathy demonstrate a 54% to 73% reduction in maximal force of muscle contraction in response to isoproterenol compared to those in normal hearts. Surprisingly, heart muscles from the same cardiomyopathy patients exhibit a force similar to normal hearts following direct stimulation by c-AMP and calcium (via histamine).[14] This suggests that some patients with dilated cardiomyopathy have an intact force generation mechanism but lack adequate signalling from β-receptor stimulation.

☑ *Catecholamines increase cardiac force by increasing delivery and reuptake of intracellular calcium.*

The Vascular Smooth Muscle Cell

Arterioles are 15-30 μm diameter branches of the vascular tree that are the site of the greatest pressure decrease and hydraulic resistance to blood flow within the circulation.[15] Smooth muscle cells that surround the circumference of each arteriole vessel wall control the diameter of these vessels. Since fluid resistance is proportional to $1/(radius)^4$, small changes in vessel size due to changes in the tone of these vascular smooth muscle cells are important dynamic determinants of resistance to blood flow.

FACTORS THAT INFLUENCE THE VASCULAR SMOOTH MUSCLE CELL CONTRACTION[16]

Vascular endothelial cells line the lumen of the arteriole wall. These cells couple changes in local lumen conditions to adjacent vascular smooth muscle cells by producing biochemical agents that affect vascular smooth muscle tone (for example, nitric oxide and endothelins). In addition, sympathetic neurotransmitters (for example, norepinephrine), circulating vasoactive hormones (for example, angiotensin II), and pharmacologically active drugs (for example, nitroprusside) all converge on the vascular smooth muscle to control arteriole diameter.

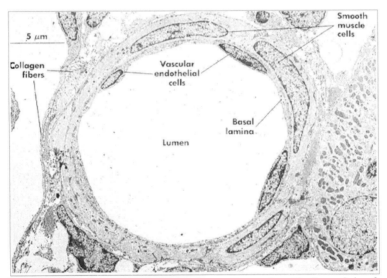

Figure 5-9. *Vascular endothelial and smooth muscle cells.* From Schauf, Charles. Human Physiology, Foundations and Frontiers. Times Mirror/Mosby College Publishing, 1990, page 355. Reproduced with permission of The McGraw-Hill Companies.[6]

VASCULAR SMOOTH MUSCLE CELL STRUCTURE

Actin and myosin contractile proteins similar to those that effect cardiac and skeletal muscle cell contraction also mediate vascular smooth muscle cell tone. Instead of a precise sarcomere array of contractile proteins, however, the smooth muscle cell has a loose arrangement of actin and myosin filaments.

☑ *Compared to cardiac muscle cells, smooth muscle cells contain a relatively large number of actin molecules.*

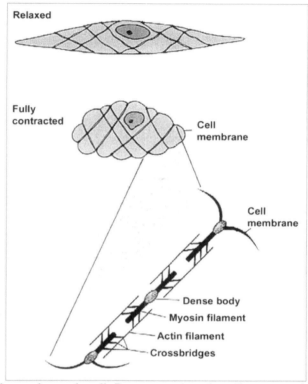

Figure 5-10. *Top — Relaxed smooth muscle cell. Bottom — when the cell contracts, it reduces vessel diameter.* From Schauf, Charles. Human Physiology, Foundations and Frontiers. Times Mirror/Mosby College Publishing, 1990, page 355. Reproduced with permission of The McGraw-Hill Companies.[6]

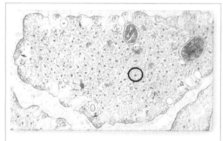

Whereas there are two cardiac actin filaments for each myosin filament, many more vascular actin filaments are present around an individual myosin filament. In this electron micrograph a single smooth muscle cell myosin filament is the center of a small circle containing dozens of surrounding actin filaments.[16]

Figure 5-11. *Electron micrograph of smooth muscle cell.* From Somlyo AP and Somlyo AV. Smooth muscle structure and function. In: Fozzard HA, Haber E, Jennings RB, Katz AM, Morgan HE, editors. The heart and cardiovascular system: Scientific foundations. 2 ed. New York: Raven Press, 1986: 847. Printed with permission of the copyright holder, Lippincott, Williams, and Wilkins.[16]

Relationship between Force and Calcium Concentration in the Smooth Muscle Cell

The relationship between force and calcium concentration in the vascular smooth muscle cell is analogous to that in the cardiac myocyte; however, the time course and mechanisms are different.[17] Following electrical depolarization (arrow), a calcium ion "pulse" (lower trace, c/s) initiates vascular smooth muscle cell force of contraction (upper trace, mg) that is manifest over minutes rather than a fraction of a second.

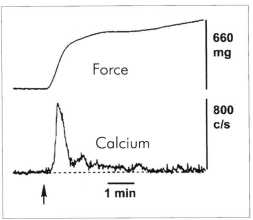

Figure 5-12. *Relationship between force and calcium concentration in the vascular smooth muscle cell.* Reprinted from the American Journal of Medicine, volume 77 , Morgan JP and Morgan KG, Calcium and cardiovascular function. Intracellular calcium levels during contraction and relaxation of mammalian cardiac and vascular smooth muscle as detected with aequorin. Page 44, Copyright 1984, with permission from Excerpta Media Inc.[17]

☑ *Intracellular calcium controls force in both heart and vascular muscle cells, but by different mechanisms.*

VASCULAR SMOOTH MUSCLE CELL CONTRACTION

Calcium channels affected by membrane protein phosphorylation control entry of calcium into the vascular smooth muscle cell. Calcium and the regulatory protein, calmodulin (CAM), activate myosin light chain kinase (MLCK). Activated MLCK with

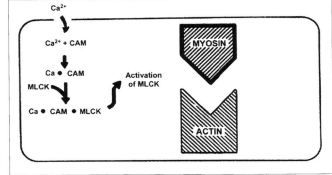

Figure 5-13. *Activation sequence of MLCK.*

ATP can phosphorylate the myosin light chain and so allow the myosin head to form crossbridges with the abundant surrounding actin filaments. Myosin activation is not required in the cardiac cell (see Chapter 6, Sarcomere).[16]

☑ *In smooth muscle cells, calcium controls <u>myosin</u> activation; In cardiac muscle cells, calcium controls <u>actin</u> activation.*

Comparison of c-AMP Pathways to Increase Cardiac Contractility and Vascular Vasodilation

Hormonal stimulation or drug interventions that increase intracellular c-AMP lead to increases in contractility in the heart and vasodilation in the vascular tree. The effects of an increase in the second messenger, c-AMP, relate to the *specific proteins* that are phosphorylated by c-AMP dependent enzymes or protein kinases in each cell.[18]

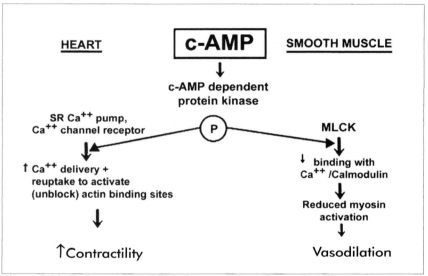

Figure 5-14. *Pathways of c-AMP in heart and smooth muscle cells.*

☑ *Increased intracellular c-AMP leads to an increase in cardiac contractility and a decrease in vascular tone.*

EFFECTS OF INCREASED c-AMP IN CARDIAC VS. SMOOTH MUSCLE CELL

In the cardiac myocyte, increased c-AMP leads to increases in calcium delivery and reuptake and to an increase in contractility. In the vascular smooth muscle cell, increased c-AMP leads to decreased binding affinity of myosin light chain kinase (MLCK) with calcium and calmodulin, resulting in vasodilation.[16]

CONTROL PATHWAY FOR C-AMP

Increased levels of c-AMP can occur either through activation of the cell membrane β-adrenergic receptor or through decreased breakdown through pharmacologic inhibition of its specific phosphodiesterase (PDE) hydrolysis enzyme.

In heart failure, despite high levels of circulating norepinephrine, myocyte concentrations of c-AMP may be low because of a down regulation in the number and activity of cell membrane adrenergic β-receptors.[13]

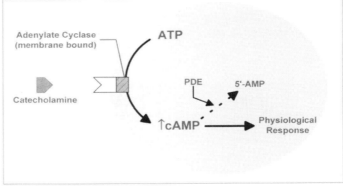

Figure 5-15. *Control pathway for c-AMP.*

CONTROL PATHWAY FOR C-GMP

Compared to c-AMP, c-GMP is present at lower concentrations within myocytes and vascular smooth muscle cells.[19] Activation of guanylate cyclase (for example, by the endothelium derived relaxing factor, nitric oxide) leads to phosphorylation by specific c-GMP dependent protein kinases.

In a vascular smooth muscle cell this will result in a decrease in intracellular calcium concentration and thus vasodilation. In a myocyte, increased formation of c-GMP can have a negative inotropic effect by decreasing calcium release into the cell during systole. Nitric oxide provides a local signal to control blood flow distribution compared to the systemic control by sympathetic nervous system activation.

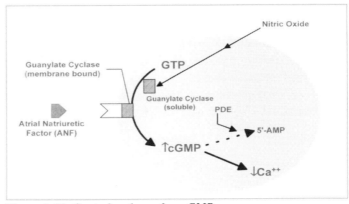

Figure 5-16. *Control pathway for c-GMP.*

Chapter 5 Quiz

1. Match the following myocyte component to its respective function:
   _____ myofibril
   _____ mitochondria
   _____ nucleus
   _____ sarcoplasmic reticulum
   _____ T-tubules
   _____ sarcolemma
   _____ lysosomes
   _____ sarcoplasm (cytoplasm)

   a. Intracellular digestion and proteolysis
   b. Provides cytosol in which rise and fall of ionized calcium occurs;
       contains other ions, small molecules, and proteins
   c. Interaction of thick and thin filaments during contraction cycle.
   d. Takes up and releases Ca^{++} during contraction cycle
   e. Provide high energy ATP chiefly for contraction and homeostasis
   f. Transmission of electrical signal from sarcolemma to cell interior
   g. mRNA synthesis
   h. Control of ionic gradients

2. The heart functions as a circulatory pump by conversion of pressure-volume work to biochemical energy and the utilization of ATP by actin and myosin.
   a) True
   b) False

3. Because of the LaPlace relationship, resting energy utilization per gram of heart tissue of the dilated failing heart is greater than the normal heart.
   a) True
   b) False

4. Complete the following equation:
   $$\frac{\text{ENERGY UTILIZATION}}{\text{GRAM OF HEART MUSCLE}} \quad \alpha \quad \text{SYSTOLIC WALL STRESS} \cdot \underline{\quad\quad}$$
   a) end-diastolic pressure
   b) heart rate
   c) stroke volume
   d) cardiac output

5. Which of the following best describes the myocyte electromechanical interval?
    a) calcium release → depolarization of electrical action potential → force generation
    b) calcium release → force generation → depolarization of electrical action potential
    c) depolarization of electrical action potential → force generation → calcium release
    d) depolarization of electrical action potential → calcium release → force generation

6. What is the relationship between the level of calcium in the papillary muscle to the generation of force?
    a) $(Ca^{++})^2 \alpha$ 1–Force
    b) $Ca^{+-} \alpha$ 1/Force
    c) $Ca^{++} \alpha$ Force
    d) $1/Ca^{++} \alpha$ Force

7. All of the following factors influence vascular smooth muscle cell contraction except:
    a) pharmacologically active drugs
    b) circulating vasoactive hormones
    c) nitric oxide
    d) superoxide dismutase

8. Increasing the levels of intracellular c-AMP has which of the following effects on the cardiac and smooth muscles?
    a) increase in cardiac contractility and smooth muscle cell vasoconstriction
    b) increase in cardiac contractility and smooth muscle cell vasodilation
    c) decrease in cardiac contractility and smooth muscle cell vasoconstriction
    d) decrease in cardiac contractility and smooth muscle cell vasodilatiation

9. In heart failure, despite high levels of circulating norepinephrine, myocyte concentrations of c-AMP may be low because of a down regulation in the number and activity of cell membrane adrenergic β-receptors.
    a) True
    b) False

                                    See Appendix for solutions.

Sarcomere

Chapter 6

This chapter provides a brief overview of the biochemical basis of sarcomere contraction and relaxation. Abnormalities in sarcomeric structure and function can result in manifestations of heart failure.

Sarcomere Structure

Within each myocyte cell, repeating units of sarcomeres arranged in series form myofibrils. Overlapping actin (thin) and myosin (thick) filaments compose the sarcomeric band pattern. A sarcomere unit, 1.5–2.5 μm in length, is the region between two adjacent Z lines (Z). Although Z lines are visible by light microscopy, the sarcomere is better seen by electron microscopy as shown here. Actin filaments project from each Z line toward the central M line (M). Myosin filaments are anchored to the central M line.[1] In heart failure, despite increases in heart chamber and cell size, sarcomere unit size remains normal.

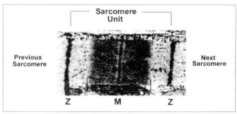

Figure 6-1. *Structure of the sarcomere.*[2] See below for permissions.

SARCOMERE CHANGES WITH MUSCLE CONTRACTION

The myosin band remains at constant length during muscular contraction, but Z lines and associated actin filaments move closer together during contraction and further apart during relaxation. The force-length characteristics of the sarcomere underlie the pressure-volume relationships of the intact ventricle.[2]

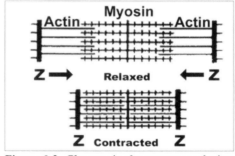

Figure 6-2. *Changes in the sarcomere during muscle contraction.*[2] See below for permissions.

MYOSIN HEAD AND TAIL ORIENTATION

The myosin molecule orients its tails toward the center of the sarcomere M line and its heads laterally. Aggregates of myosin molecules form a thick myofilament.[2]

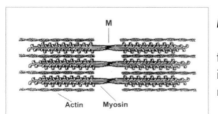

Figure 6-3. *Myosin head and tail orientation.*[2] Figures 6-1, 6-2, and 6-3 from Ganong WF. Excitable tissue: muscle. In: Review of medical physiology. 17th ed. Norwalk: Appleton & Lange, 1995:57-58. Permission granted by the copyright holder: Lippincott, Willams and Wilkins.

Myosin Structure

Hundreds of myosin proteins aggregate within each thick filament of the sarcomere. A myosin protein consists of two heavy chain subunits each with a globular head and a long tail. Two myosin light chains bind to each heavy chain subunit. Myosin globular heads bind to neighboring actin molecules to form crossbridges along the entire length of the actin filament. The myocyte can synthesize alternate isoforms of myosin in response to changes in metabolic state. For instance, in hyperthyroid states, a "fast" myosin will predominate with faster contraction and higher utilization of ATP and oxygen.[1]

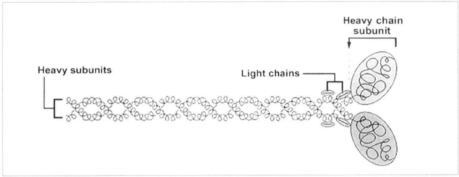

Figure 6-4. *Myosin structure.* From Katz AM. Physiology of the heart. Raven Press, New York, 1992; 153. Permission granted by the copyright holders: Arnold Katz and Lippincott, Willams and Wilkins.[3]

Actin Structure

The thin filament of the sarcomere is a double helix created by repeating units of actin. Tropomyosin fits into grooves of the actin thin filament. Troponin is a regulatory three-component protein dispersed along the tropomyosin filament composed of troponin T that binds to tropomyosin, troponin I that controls the myosin binding site on actin, and troponin C that includes regulatory sites for calcium binding.[1]

Levosimendan is an example of a new class of cardiac inotropic drugs, calcium sensitizers, which act by binding to troponin C. By doing so, they increase the force generated for any concentration of intracellular calcium.[4]

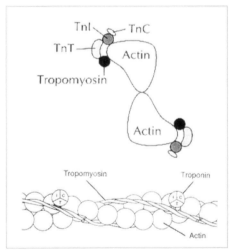

Figure 6-5. *Actin structure.* From Katz AM. Physiology of the heart. Raven Press, New York, 1992; 166. Permission granted by the copyright holders: Arnold Katz and Lippincott, Willams and Wilkins.[3]

Activation of Contraction

The action potential initiates the influx of calcium into the myocyte and the release of calcium from intracellular stores within the sarcoplasmic reticulum. When calcium binds to troponin C, a conformational change occurs within the troponin trimer which displaces tropomyosin and exposes the actin binding site to permit the formation of an actin-myosin crossbridge.[1]

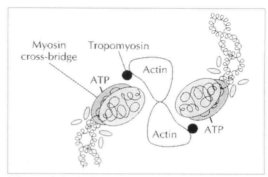

Figure 6-6. *Actin-myosin crossbridge formation.* From Katz AM. Physiology of the heart. Raven Press, New York, 1992; 181. Permission granted by the copyright holders: Arnold Katz and Lippincott, Willams and Wilkins.[3]

The Power Stroke

The power stroke produces muscular contraction. Chemical energy derived from ATP hydrolysis bends the myosin head by closing an open cleft as it binds to actin. Actin and myosin filaments slide past each other producing a "power stroke." Each myosin head may repeat this power stroke during a single systolic contraction. The stored energy is released when the myosin head straightens to return to its native position.[2]

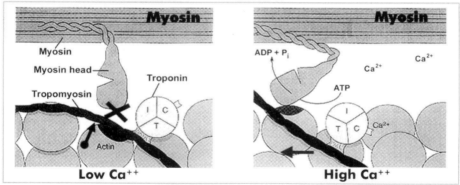

Figure 6-7. *The power stroke.*[2] From Ganong WF. Excitable tissue: muscle. In: Review of medical physiology. 17 th ed. Norwalk: Appleton & Lange, 1995:57-58. Permission granted by the copyright holder: Lippincott, Willams and Wilkins.

MUSCLE RELAXATION

Following myocyte electrical repolarization, increased intracellular calcium returns to the sarcoplasmic reticulum via ATP dependent active transport in preparation for the next contractile cycle. Thus, calcium movement provides the signal and ATP hydrolysis provides the energy for both contraction and relaxation.

Chapter 6 Quiz

1. The myosin band of the sarcomere moves closer together during contraction and further apart during relaxation, while the Z lines remain constant throughout both processes.
   - a) True
   - b) False

2. The myosin molecule orients its head toward the center of the sarcomere M line and its tail laterally. Aggregates of myosin molecules form a thick myofilament.
   - a) True
   - b) False

3. The myosin protein is composed of:
   - a) 4 subunits – 3 heavy and 1 light chains
   - b) 4 subunits – 1 heavy and 3 light chains
   - c) 6 subunits – 2 heavy and 4 light chains
   - d) 6 subunits – 4 heavy and 2 light chains

4. All of the following is true of the troponin protein except:
   - a) it is a regulatory protein
   - b) it fits into the grooves of the myosin thick filament
   - c) it has 3 components: T, which binds to tropomyosin; I, which controls the myosin biding site on actin; and C, which includes the regulatory sites for calcium binding
   - d) all of the above

5. The action potential initiates the influx of calcium into the myocyte and the release of calcium from intracellular stores within the sarcoplasmic reticulum. Which of the following best describes the subsequent steps in the contractile process?
   - a) conformational change in troponin trimer → binding of Ca^{++} to troponin C → displacement of tropomyosin → formation of actin-myosin crossbridge → exposure of actin binding site
   - b) conformational change in troponin trimer → displacement of tropomyosin → binding of Ca^{++} to troponin C → formation of actin-myosin crossbridge → exposure of actin binding site

c) binding of Ca^{++} to troponin C → exposure of actin
binding site → conformational change in troponin trimer
→ displacement of tropomyosin → formation of actin-
myosin crossbridge

d) binding of Ca^{++} to troponin C → conformational change
in troponin trimer → displacement of tropomyosin →
exposure of actin binding site → formation of actin-myosin
crossbridge

6. All of the following events occur in the power stroke for muscle contraction except:

a) No energy is required for calcium reuptake and muscle
relaxation

b) each myosin head may repeat the power stroke during a
single systolic contraction

c) actin and myosin filaments slide past each other

d) chemical energy derived from ATP hydrolysis bends the
myosin head by closing an open cleft as it binds to actin

See Appendix for solutions.

Gene

Chapter 7

A molecular biology view of heart failure identifies various mechanisms of cardiac remodeling and apoptosis. This chapter looks at the role of the gene in the progression of heart failure.

Signal Transduction Pathways for Cardiac Myocyte Hypertrophy

TRIGGERS OF HYPERTROPHY

Accompanied by changes in heart fibroblasts and vascular structures, cardiac myocyte hypertrophy is a dominant mechanism of change in heart structure and size. Cytokine growth factors (protein mediators of intercellular signaling and inflammation), vasoactive hormones, and myocyte stretch or increased wall stress are all known triggers of myocyte hypertrophy. These factors stimulate a cascade of phosphorylation of intracellular proteins that ultimately activate protein transcription factors within the nucleus. By binding to DNA, transcription factors initiate the creation of RNA transcripts that lead to the enlargement of the ventricles.[1]

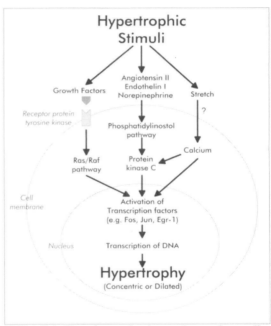

Figure 7-1. *Signal transduction pathways for cardiac hypertrophy.*[1]

In heart failure, heart size affects patient outcome. For example, Lee, et al found that increasing heart size measured by echocardiographic left ventricular internal diastolic dimension predicted mortality in patients with advanced heart failure.[2]

Evidence of Apoptosis in Heart Failure

Loss of functioning myocytes is a characteristic of heart failure due to systolic dysfunction.[3,4] Recently, programmed cell death or apoptosis has been recognized to be a significant contributing factor to cell loss distinct from necrosis secondary to ischemic or other injury. Compared to necrosis, apoptosis is an energy requiring process with a characteristic fragmentation of chromosomal DNA usually without inflammatory cell infiltrates.[5] Adaptive or maladaptive ventricular remodeling will occur as a cumulative effect of both cell hypertrophy and cell death.

> ☑ *Biochemical signals that promote cell growth in some cells may lead to cell death and apoptosis in others.[6]*

In a study of asymptomatic immediate family members of patients with idiopathic dilated cardiomyopathy, 25% had left ventricular enlargement by echocardiography. Five of these asymptomatic individuals underwent heart biopsy. All five had evidence of apoptosis and abnormal cell surface protein expression without overt inflammation.[7] This suggests a primary role of apoptosis in some patients with dilated cardiomyopathy.

Olivetti and coworkers detected heart muscle cell chromosome breakage typical of apoptosis by nuclear binding of the fluorescent artificial nucleotide deoxyuridine triphosphate. Although failing hearts showed evidence of scarring due to necrosis, hearts from both ischemic and idiopathic dilated cardiomyopathy also had an approximately 240-fold increase in the fraction of myocytes undergoing apoptosis compared to hearts from control individuals dying without cardiovascular disease. In the future, acute or chronic therapy to prevent myocardial cell loss due to apoptosis may complement strategies tailored to blunt hypertrophy and necrosis.

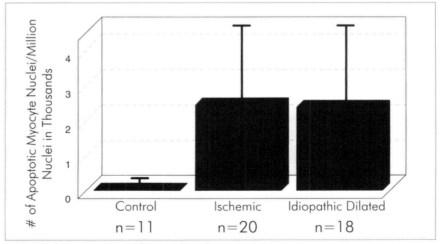

Figure 7-2. *Apoptosis and heart failure.[5]*

Animal Model of Apoptosis

CHANGES DURING THE TRANSITION FROM STABLE HYPERTROPHY TO HEART FAILURE IN SPONTANEOUSLY HYPERTENSIVE RATS

The loss of viable myocytes may contribute to progressive deterioration of left ventricular function. Activation of intracellular protein myocyte growth factors (proto-oncogenes), such as c-myc and c-fos, can lead to both the acceleration of protein synthesis and the initiation of apoptosis. Extracellular fibrosis replaces myocytes eliminated by apoptosis. Both may contribute to remodelling of the heart.[8]

EXPERIENCE WITH SPONTANEOUSLY HYPERTENSIVE RATS

Spontaneously hypertensive rats exhibit the transition from normal to stable hypertrophy to progressive signs of heart failure, including left ventricular dilatation and decreased ejection fraction. Assessment of percent myocardial fibrosis in this animal model of heart failure illustrates the possible role of apoptosis in the pathogenesis of heart failure. Heart failure rats have the highest fibrosis fractional area with the lowest myocyte fractional area compared to both normal rats and rats with stable hypertrophy prior to the development of heart failure.[9]

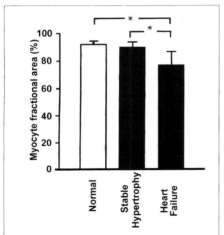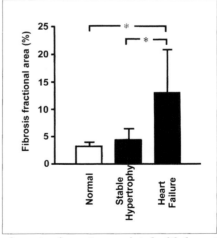

Figure 7-3. *Heart failure in spontaneously hypertensive rats associated with loss of myocytes and replacement with fibrosis.* Reprinted from the European Heart Journal, Vol 16 (Suppl N). Boluyt MO, Bing OH, Lakatta EG. The ageing spontaneously hypertensive rat as a model of the transition from stable compensated hypertrophy to heart failure, page 21, 1995, by permission of the publisher: WB Saunders Company Limited.[9]

Inducible Tumor Necrosis Factor-α (TNF-α) in Patients with Dilated Cardiomyopathy

The heart is the *target* for a spectrum of cytokines that can depress heart function and act as growth factors contributing to ventricular enlargement. However, in advanced heart failure the heart can be a *source* of these cytokines that act locally or systemically. The expression of a new and deleterious repertoire of cytokines may contribute to the downward spiral of advanced heart failure.[10] Tumor necrosis factor, normally produced primarily by monocytes, can act as a myocardial depressant factor and systemically lead to anorexia and cachexia.[11] Satoh and colleagues detected TNF-α messenger RNA by Northern blot analysis in cardiac biopsies from19 of 25 patients with dilated cardiomyopathy localized to myocytes and endomyocardial endothelium. No TNF-α messenger RNA was detected in biopsies from control patients without heart failure.[12] Recently, administration of an intravenous genetically engineered soluble binder of TNF-α to12 patients with heart failure led to an improvement in measured quality of life scores, six-minute walk distance, and ejection fraction.[13]

☑ *Pharmacologic blockade of the cytokine TNF-α may be an important heart failure therapy in the future.*

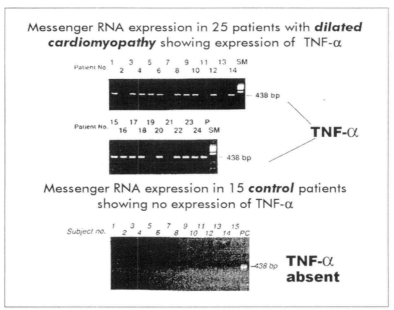

Figure 7-4. *Messenger RNA expression of TNF-α in patients with cardiomyopathy vs. control patients.* Adapted with permission from the American College of Cardiology (Journal of the American College of Cardiology, March 1997; 29:719).[12]

Chapter 7 Quiz

1. Heart size is a predictor of outcome in patients with heart failure.
    a) True
    b) False

2. Which of the following are considered to be *triggers* of myocyte hypertrophy:
    a) cytokine growth factors
    b) vasoactive hormones
    c) increased wall stress
    d) all of the above

3. Which of the following is not involved in the pathway for activating transcription factors in cardiac muscle hypertrophy?
    a) angiotensin I
    b) endothelin I
    c) growth factors
    d) norepinephrine

4. Apoptosis is an energy requiring process with characteristic fragmentation of chromosomal DNA which occurs usually without the presence of inflammatory cell infiltrates.
    a) True
    b) False

5. Rats with heart failure have significantly _____ fibrosis fractional areas and _____ myocyte fractional areas compared to normal rats.
    a) less; greater
    b) greater; less
    c) greater; greater
    d) less; less

6. The myocyte is a source, rather than a target, for a spectrum of
   cytokines that depress heart function and contribute to ventricular
   enlargement.

      a) True

      b) False

See Appendix for solutions.

Molecule
Chapter 8

A research goal of cardiovascular medicine is to understand the molecular basis of heart failure with the aim of developing new heart failure therapies. In this chapter, molecular investigation in heart failure is introduced.

Hypertrophic Cardiomyopathy

One molecular cause of heart failure, hypertrophic cardiomyopathy, has a dominant pattern of inheritance with variable penetrance (see page 128). Common abnormalities (approximately 35%) occur because of a single amino acid substitution within the myosin heavy chain head. Other identified genetic defects include those that lead to amino acid changes within the myosin-binding protein C, the control protein, troponin, and other proteins within the sarcomeric unit. Some patients with genetic causes of hypertrophic cardiomyopathy may be difficult to identify since the abnormal hypertrophied ventricle phenotype may not be manifest until after age 60.[1]

Why amino acid substitutions in these different areas lead to the full spectrum of hypertrophic changes including histologic disorganization of myocytes within the ventricular wall, asymmetric septal hypertrophy, and cardiac arrhythmias is not fully known at this time. Nevertheless, the identification of these specific defects contributes to the hope that future therapies can be identified to correct them.[2]

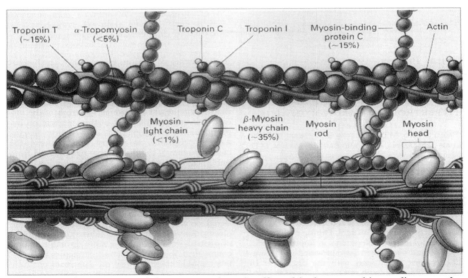

Figure 8-1. *Components of the sarcomeric unit affected in hypertrophic cardiomyopathy.* Reprinted with permission from The New England Journal of Medicine, copyright © 1997 Massachusetts Medical Society. All rights reserved. (New England Journal of Medicine, March 1997:336:775-785).[2]

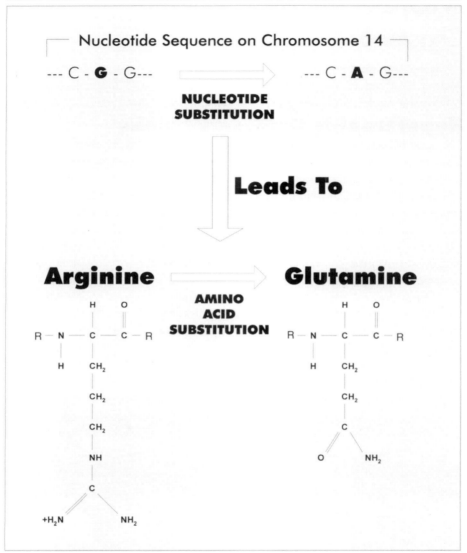

Figure 8-2. *Example of missense mutation in the long arm of chromosome 14 coding for β-myosin heavy chain leading to an arginine to glutamine substitution. This amino acid substitution leads to a form of hypertrophic cardiomyopathy with an increased risk of sudden death.*[3]

☑ *A form of hypertrophic cardiomyopathy with an increased risk of sudden death is caused by a missense mutation leading to a glutamine for arginine substitution in the longarm of chromosome 14.*[3]

Effects of Phospholamban Phosphorylation on the Calcium Pump of the Cardiac Sarcoplasmic Reticulum

Catecholamine stimulation of the myocyte increases intracellular c-AMP. A step in the transduction of this signal into a change in inotropic state occurs with the phosphorylation of the inhibiting protein, phospholamban, bound to the pump protein Sarco(endo) plasmic reticulum calcium ATPase (SERCA-2) (see page 73). When phospholamban is phosphorylated (note large arrow in Figure 8-3) it permits a greater active transport of calcium from the lower concentration cytoplasm to the higher concentration sarcoplasmic reticulum.[4]

Patients with heart failure may have reduced synthesis of both the phospholamban as well as the calcium ATPase pump proteins which may reduce maximum force generation with electrical depolarization.[5]

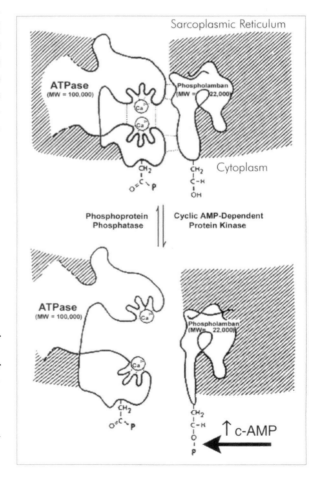

Figure 8-3. *Schematic representation of the effects of phospholamban phosphorylation on the calcium pump of the cardiac sarcoplasmic reticulum.* Reprinted with permission from The American College of Cardiology (Journal of the American College of Cardiology, 1983:1:42-51).[4]

Chapter 8 Quiz

1. Which of the following has a dominant pattern of inheritance with variable penetrance?

    a) dilated cardiomyopathy

    b) idiopathic cardiomyopathy

    c) hypertrophic cardiomyopathy

    d) viral cardiomyopathy

2. All of the following are known genetic abnormalities that may lead to heart failure except:

    a) a single amino acid substitution within the myosin heavy chain head

    b) a frameshift mutation within the actin-myosin binding site

    c) amino acid changes within the myosin-binding protein C

    d) amino acid changes with the control protein troponin within the sarcomeric unit

3. Patients with heart failure may have reduced synthesis of both the phospholamban as well as the calcium ATPase pump proteins which may reduce force generation with electrical depolarization.

    a) True

    b) False

See Appendix for solutions.

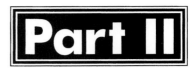

Part II

The Management of Heart Failure

Diagnosis

Chapter 9

Part II, The Management of Heart Failure, divides heart failure management into three categories — Diagnosis, Outpatient Therapy, and Inpatient Therapy. Case scenarios at the end of each chapter present a problem based approach to treating heart failure patients. Throughout Part II, emphasis is placed on multicenter trials that serve as guides in treating the heart failure patient.

The initial chapter of Part II, Diagnosis, provides a three-step process of evaluating patients — leading to an accurate diagnosis of the patient with heart failure.

Assessment of Heart Failure

Caring for your patient with heart failure requires repetition of a clinical cycle of assessment, initiation of a clinical plan, and reassessment. Especially if new symptoms occur, you should determine if they fit the diagnosis of heart failure, if the original diagnosis of heart failure is still systolic, diastolic, or other dysfunction, and if there are new treatable, causes of heart failure present.

THREE-STEP ASSESSMENT OF HEART FAILURE:

1. **DOES PRESENTATION FIT THE DIAGNOSIS OF HEART FAILURE?**

2. **IS SYSTOLIC OR DIASTOLIC LV FUNCTION ABNORMAL?**

3. **ARE THERE TREATABLE CAUSES OF HEART FAILURE PRESENT?**

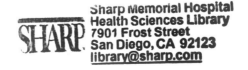

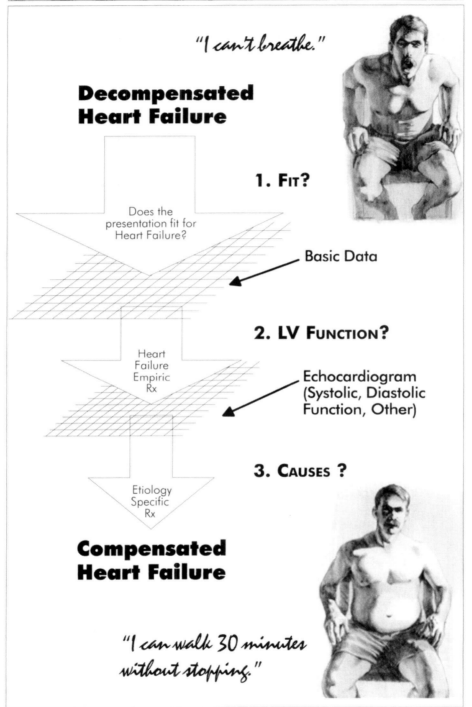

Figure 9-1. *Three-step assessment of heart failure.* Illustrations by Peter Chapman.

Step 1:
Does Presentation Fit the Diagnosis of Heart Failure?

Even an experienced clinician can miss the diagnosis of heart failure. Preexisting chronic obstructive lung disease or renal insufficiency can obscure the etiology of shortness of breath or fatigue. Shortness of breath in a young person due to either cardiomyopathy or myocarditis is often attributed to asthma or pneumonitis.

Conversely, when a patient has a history of heart failure, the diverse manifestations of this syndrome may mislead you into thinking that all symptoms are due to heart failure rather than to a new alternative diagnosis.

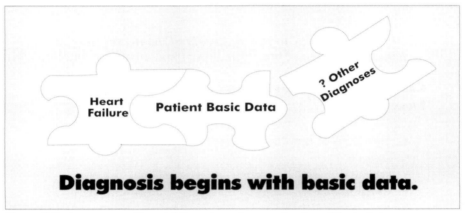

Figure 9-2. *Assessment of heart failure depends on evaluation of basic data.*

Characteristic initial history and physical exam findings should lead you to look further. Very few patients have symptoms due to heart failure with a normal ECG and chest x-ray. A chest x-ray may show cardiomegaly or bilateral pulmonary infiltrates consistent with edema.

☑ *Patients with heart failure usually have an abnormal ECG, chest x-ray, or both.*

Basic Data
• History and Physical Exam
• Lab: Chem 20, CBC, Urinalysis
• Electrocardiogram (ECG)
• Chest x-ray (CXR)

If an empiric trial of diuretics leads to improvement, pulmonary congestion due to heart failure is likely, especially if echo-Doppler abnormalities are present (see Step 2). Alternatively, when nonspecific interstitial infiltrates are present on chest x-ray, patients may require measurement of pulmonary capillary wedge pressure to distinguish heart failure from pulmonary infection or fibrosis.

HISTORY

The history is the first step to determine if patient symptoms fit the diagnosis of heart failure. You should attempt to address the following cardinal symptoms in the history for possible heart failure in all patients. It is important to recall that these cardinal symptoms, although consistent with the diagnosis of heart failure, can also have alternate etiologies.

☑ *History is the key to the diagnosis of the presence of heart failure.*

CARDINAL SYMPTOMS IN HISTORY FOR POSSIBLE HEART FAILURE

- Shortness of breath (when active or recumbent)
- Fatigue
- Edema
- Chest pain

ALTERNATE ETIOLOGIES OF CARDINAL SYMPTOMS

Shortness of Breath	Fatigue
• Pulmonary	• Anemia
• Anemia	• Musculoskeletal
• Musculoskeletal	• Metabolic
• Functional	• Functional
Edema	**Chest Pain**
• Renal	• Gastrointestinal
• Hepatic	• Pulmonary
• Nutritional	• Musculoskeletal
• Venous insufficiency	• Functional

☑ *When evaluating a patient for possible heart failure, also consider pulmonary, musculoskeletal, anemia, and functional causes of shortness of breath as alternative diagnoses.*

PAST MEDICAL HISTORY

Does the patient have previously known medical problems that could contribute to heart failure?
- Myocardial infarction
- Coronary Artery Disease
- Hypertension
- Diabetes mellitus
- Thyroid disease
- Cardiotoxic chemotherapy
- Autoimmune disease
- Severe viral illness
- Rheumatic Fever as a child

Does the patient have risk factors for coronary artery disease such as hypertension, hyperlipidemia, smoking, and diabetes mellitus?

☑ *Coronary artery disease, hypertension, and diabetes are common preexisting conditions that may be associated with heart failure.*

FAMILY HISTORY
- Is there a family history of heart failure or coronary artery disease?
- Is there a family history of early unexplained or sudden death?

☑ *Familial cardiomyopathy may be previously unrecognized.*

SOCIAL HISTORY
- Is alcohol use excessive?
- Is there a history of illicit drug use?
- Is there an adequate family or social support structure?
- Has there been any unusual travel and/or exposure (e.g. animals)?

☑ *Toxic cardiomyopathy due to alcohol or drugs can be a sole or contributing cause of heart failure.*

PHYSICAL EXAM

Surprisingly, when we see individuals with ventricular dysfunction, most will appear completely comfortable at rest and with simple ambulation. Only with physical exertion or decompensated heart failure, do patients appear overtly short of breath or fatigued.

VITAL SIGNS

- Is the patient hyper- or hypotensive?

Measurement of blood pressure and heart rate are important findings from the physical exam in a patient with either compensated or decompensated heart failure. Hypertension indicates a need for additional vasodilator, β-blocker, or diuretic therapy.

> ☑ *In a previously healthy individual, fever and hypotension*
> *followed by pulmonary edema with intravenous hydration*
> *is a presentation of severe myocarditis.*

- Is pulse pressure reduced?

A patient's proportional pulse pressure correlates with their cardiac index (see page 20).

- Is the patient's heart rate normal, increased, or decreased?

Any rapid atrial arrhythmia may lead to heart failure if sustained for a long period of time. Sinus tachycardia often implies a low reserve with activity associated with a reduced stroke volume and associated small pulse pressure. Conversely, bradycardia (heart rate less than 50 beats per minute associated with heart block) may be a reason for heart failure. Resting heart rate also indicates if β-blocker therapy will lead to symptomatic bradycardia.

> ☑ *Sustained supraventricular tachycardia is a treatable*
> *cause of cardiomyopathy.*

- Is the patient "wet" or "dry"?

After measurement of vital signs, a goal of the physical exam is to determine if a patient is "wet" (volume overloaded) or "dry" (intravascularly depleted). Criteria for heart failure include jugular venous neck vein distention, rales, S_3 gallop, abdominojugular reflux, hepatomegaly, and peripheral edema. Any of these findings can indicate elevated ventricular filling pressures or that the patient is "wet." Physical exam findings including an orthostatic decrease in blood pressure or decreased skin turgor can support the finding that a patient has intravascular depletion or is "dry." More commonly this is suggested by the findings of weight loss, history of a gastrointestinal syndrome, or laboratory evidence of an increased BUN to creatinine ratio.

☑ *The window of compensation between "wet" and "dry" gradually narrows as the degree of heart failure progresses.*

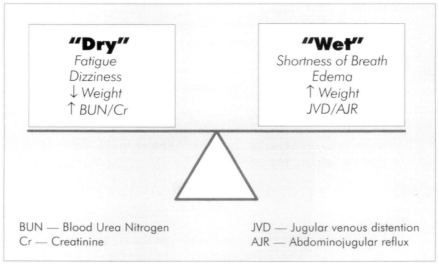

Figure 9-3. *Assessing if patients are "wet" or "dry."*

LABORATORY TESTS

Chemistry

BLOOD UREA NITROGEN (BUN)/CREATININE (CR):

Increased BUN and creatinine are consistent with inadequate renal perfusion or intrinsic renal disease.

BILIRUBIN, SGOT/SGPT, ALKALINE PHOSPHATASE/GGT

Abnormal liver function tests may indicate passive congestion with right heart failure, primary hepatic dysfunction, or both.

SODIUM (NA⁺)

Low serum Na^+ concentration indicates high neurohormonal activation associated with high arginine vasopressin (ADH) and angiotensin II levels.

POTASSIUM (K⁺)

Often decreases with diuretics, but increases with ACE inhibitors and renal insufficiency.

MAGNESIUM (MG⁺⁺)

Potentially decreased with diuretics which can contribute to arrhythmias.

TROPONIN I

A sensitive and specific indicator of myocardial infarction in acute coronary syndromes.

CBC

ANEMIA

Contributes to heart failure decompensation or high output heart failure if sustained.

Urinalysis

PROTEINUREA

Low serum protein can contribute to edema due to inadequate oncotic pressure.

☑ *Hyponatremia may indicate either volume overload or depletion. Both are common in heart failure.*

HEART FAILURE "LETHAL TRIAD"

An ominous sign is present when a patient is hypotensive, despite overt activation of the sympathetic nervous system (indicated by a heart rate > 100) and of the angiotensin system (indicated by a sodium concentration < 130). The low sodium is also important because it only occurs after a sustained deterioration. Patients with a sodium concentration less than 130 are prone to marked hypotension with initiation of ACE inhibitor therapy. Titrate carefully when this is present.

$\boxed{\checkmark}$ *Heart failure "Lethal Triad"*

$$BP_{sys} < 100$$
$$HR > 100$$
$$[Na^+] < 130$$

ECG

Abnormalities are often present on resting ECG in patients with heart failure.

Findings	Suspected Diagnosis
Acute ST-T changes	Myocardial ischemia
Atrial fibrillation, other tachyarrhythmia	Thyroid disease or heart failure due to rapid ventricular rate
Bradyarrhythmias	Heart failure due to low heart rate/heart block
Previous MI (e.g. Q waves)	Heart failure due to reduced left ventricular performance
Low voltage	Pericardial effusion, amyloidosis
Left ventricular hypertrophy	Diastolic dysfunction

Figure 9-4. *Corresponding ECG findings and suspected diagnoses.* [1]

Chest X-Ray (CXR)

- Is the cardiac silhouette enlarged? (i.e., Is a/b > 0.5?)
    - √ LV dilation
    - √ LV hypertrophy
    - √ RV enlargement (may be present on lateral film only)
    - √ Pericardial effusion

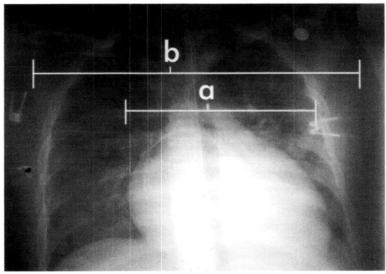

Figure 9-5. *Chest x-ray demonstrating heart failure (a/b > 0.5).*

- Are pulmonary infiltrates present?
    - √ Edema
    - √ Other causes of dyspnea (i.e., fibrosis, pneumonia, inflammation)

CXR Findings of Increased Left Heart Filling Pressure
(Left atrial and pulmonary capillary wedge pressures)
- Pulmonary venous redistribution
- Kerley B lines (horizontal interstitial lines in lateral lower lung bases)
- Perihilar infiltrates
- Pleural effusions
- Diffuse infiltrates
- Prominent azygos vein

In the patient with chronic heart failure, a chest x-ray and physical exam can be free of findings of lung congestion despite a markedly elevated pulmonary capillary wedge pressure. This may relate to chronic enlargement of lung lymphatics compensating for increased left heart filling pressures with increased return of interstitial edema to the venous system. Clear lung fields are also seen in right heart failure and in cardiomyopathy with biventricular failure.

Step 2:
LV Function — Echocardiogram

If patients have symptoms or physical exam findings suggestive of heart failure, you should obtain an echocardiogram. A majority of patients with heart failure will have a significantly reduced ejection fraction (EF) less than or equal to 40% consistent with systolic dysfunction. Multicenter trials with this finding as an entry criteria have defined evidence-based therapies for this group of patients. Nonetheless, an ejection fraction between 40 and 55% is also abnormal, but it is uncommon for this alone to result in the clinical findings of heart failure without associated diastolic dysfunction.

If you suspect diastolic dysfunction in a patient with a normal ejection fraction, look for the presence of increased LV wall thickness (left ventricular hypertrophy), left atrial enlargement, or diastolic Doppler flow abnormalities (see pages 122–127). Consider radionuclide ventriculography as an alternative test of left ventricular ejection fraction for patients who are not well imaged by echocardiography.

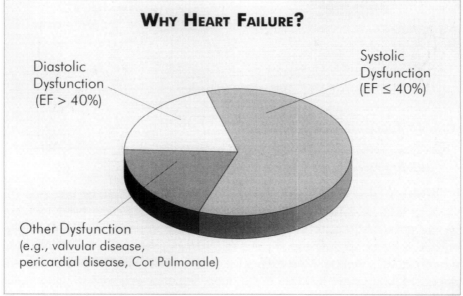

Figure 9-6. *Etiology of heart failure.*

☑ *Echocardiography is key to the diagnosis of etiology and severity of heart failure.*

Step 3:
Causes

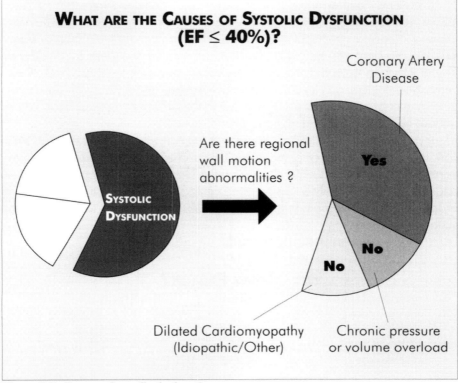

WHAT ARE THE CAUSES OF SYSTOLIC DYSFUNCTION (EF ≤ 40%)?

Coronary Artery Disease

SYSTOLIC DYSFUNCTION

Are there regional wall motion abnormalities?

Yes

No

No

Dilated Cardiomyopathy (Idiopathic/Other)

Chronic pressure or volume overload

Figure 9-7. *Causes of systolic dysfunction.*

☑ *Coronary artery disease and hypertension are the most common etiologies of heart failure.*

When an echocardiogram identifies an ejection fraction of less than or equal to 40%, by definition, the patient has systolic dysfunction. Next, look for the presence or absence of regional wall motion abnormalities that usually indicate ischemic cardiomyopathy due to coronary artery disease. Typically with ischemic cardiomyopathy, the contraction of the base of the heart is preserved compared to impaired function of the apex. Regional wall motion abnormalities that do not fit a simple vascular distribution can be found in patients with non-ischemic systolic dysfunction. In the absence of regional wall motion abnormalities, however, chronic pressure or volume overload or dilated cardiomyopathy is more likely. Dilated cardiomyopathy may be defined as primary myocardial systolic dysfunction with enlargement of the left or both ventricles in the absence of significant coronary artery disease or chronic pressure or volume overload.[2]

CORONARY ARTERY DISEASE

Coronary artery disease is a common cause of heart failure and is potentially treatable. A history of angina, myocardial infarction, or regional wall motion abnormalities on echocardiography helps identify the patient with coronary artery disease. Revascularization may lead to benefit in the presence of angina or findings of ischemia on non-invasive testing.

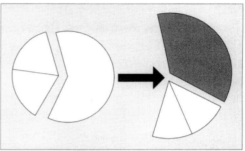

Figure 9-8. *A proportion of systolic dysfunction is attributed to coronary artery disease.*

☑ *Ischemic cardiomyopathy typically has preservation of function of the base compared to the apex of the heart.*

CHRONIC PRESSURE OR VOLUME OVERLOAD

Chronic pressure or volume overload may be a treatable cause of heart failure. Pressure overload may be secondary to systemic hypertension or aortic stenosis. Volume overload may relate to valvular regurgitation (either mitral or aortic regurgitation) or high output heart failure states such as thyrotoxicosis or chronic anemia.

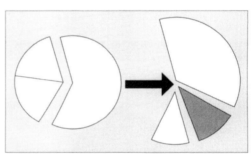

Figure 9-9. *A proportion of systolic dysfunction is attributed to chronic pressure or volume overload.*

DILATED CARDIOMYOPATHY (IDIOPATHIC/OTHER)

Finally, the presence of diffuse hypokinesis without obvious causes for pressure or volume overload, usually implies the presence of cardiomyopathy. Although non-ischemic cardiomyopathies are often idiopathic, a variety of identifiable and treatable causes exist.

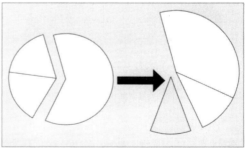

Figure 9-10. *A proportion of systolic dysfunction is attributed to dilated cardiomyopathy.*

Evaluation of the Heart Failure Patient for Myocardial Revascularization

PATIENTS WITH ANGINA OR RECURRENT ACUTE PULMONARY EDEMA

You should advise heart failure patients without contraindications to revascularization who have exercise-limiting angina, angina at rest, or recurrent episodes of acute pulmonary edema to undergo coronary artery angiography as the initial test for operable coronary lesions.

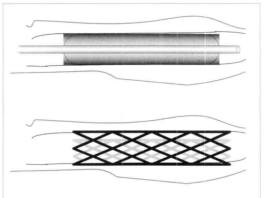

☑ *Angina usually implies the presence of viable ischemic myocardium.*

Figure 9-11. *Percutaneous revascularization via balloon angioplasty or stent.*

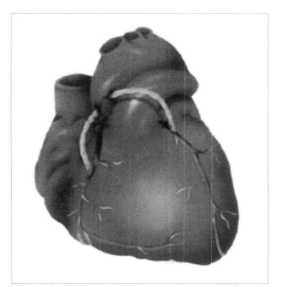

☑ *Revascularization of ischemic myocardium can lead to significant improvements in ventricular function.*

Figure 9-12. *Coronary artery bypass graft (CABG) revascularization.*

Patients with a History of Myocardial Infarction but without Significant Angina

You should recommend that these patients undergo a physiologic test for ischemia, followed by coronary angiography if ischemic regions are detected. Patients with large areas of ischemia may benefit from revascularization.

Since many patients with left ventricular dysfunction have a blunted exercise capacity, pharmacologic rather than exercise stress with adenosine (or persantine) for nuclear perfusion or dobutamine for echo wall motion is often needed. Abnormalities of perfusion can be imaged by isotope scintigraphy, such as thallium-201 (^{201}Tl), technetium-99m-sestamibi (^{99m}Tc-sestamibi) or Myoview® scanning (with rest, post-stress, and possibly rest reinjection imaging). Abnormalities of regional wall motion can be imaged by echocardiography. Positron emission tomography is an alternative imaging modality for assessing myocardial ischemia and viability, but is not widely available.

☑ *Patients with only infarcted myocardium do not benefit from revascularization.*

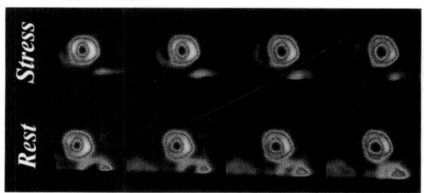

Figure 9-13. *Scintigraphy of a normal heart; notice uniform perfusion is present in both the resting and stress states.*

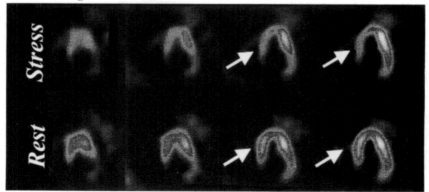

Figure 9-14. *Heart with myocardial ischemia in septal wall of left ventricle; notice the uniform perfusion in the resting state changes in the stress state (arrows).*

Useful Definitions

ISCHEMIC MYOCARDIUM

Heart muscle that functions at rest, but fails to increase in function with hemodynamic stress due to inadequate regional coronary flow reserve.

HIBERNATING MYOCARDIUM

Viable heart muscle that does not function adequately at rest due to chronically decreased oxygen supply that improves after revascularization.[3, 4]

☑ *Ischemic and hibernating myocardium may coexist in the same patient.*

Detection of hibernating myocardium predicts long-term survival after revascularization in patients with ischemic systolic disfunction heart failure.[5]

Example of Hibernating Myocardium

A patient with ischemic cardiomyopathy and significant evidence of hibernating myocardium may be a candidate for revascularization.

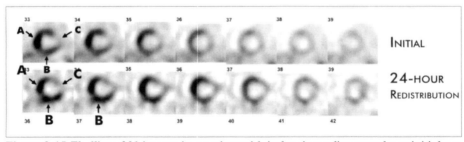

Figure 9-15. *Thallium-201 images in a patient with ischemic cardiomyopathy at initial rest and 24-hour redistribution showing normal (A), hibernating (B), and infarcted (C) zones of cardiac muscle.*

☑ *Patients with both diabetes mellitus and coronary artery disease commonly have ischemic or hibernating myocardium without symptoms of angina.*

Detecting Ischemic vs. Hibernating Myocardium

NUCLEAR SCINTIGRAPHY

- To detect ischemic myocardium associated with a decrease in regional coronary blood flow reserve use adenosine IV, persantine IV, or exercise for "stress."

- To detect hibernating myocardium, the greatest amount of data is available with ^{201}Tl uptake as indicator of viability; less data is available with ^{99m}Tc-sestamibi and Myoview.® Thallium-201 reinjection at 24-hours can further assess uptake to indicate viability.

DOBUTAMINE STRESS ECHOCARDIOGRAPHY

- To detect ischemic myocardium look for worsening of preserved wall motion with 10-40 µg/kg/min of dobutamine.

- To identify hibernating myocardium by stimulating contractile reserve, look for improvement in impaired wall motion with 5-10 µg/kg/min dobutamine. Patients with both hibernating and ischemic myocardium may have a biphasic initial improvement in wall motion followed by deterioration of wall motion.[6]

- Dobutamine can lead to a false negative for detecting viability if myocardium develops further ischemic dysfunction rather than demonstrating reserve.

- Requires adequate echocardiographic windows and images.

☑ *Patients with a biphasic response of improvement followed by worsening in myocardial contraction during dobutamine stress echocardiography may exhibit the greatest recovery of rest function after revascularization.[7]*

Nuclear Scintigraphy vs. Dobutamine Stress Echocardiography for Detecting Myocardial Ischemia

There is disagreement whether stress test assessment of perfusion by nuclear isotope scanning or ventricular wall motion by echocardiography is a better way to detect the presence of myocardial ischemia. The presence of local expertise in one of the two modalities may determine which is preferred for your patient. In general, sensitivity of detecting myocardial ischemia and validation of benefit of revascularization are slightly higher with nuclear scanning techniques. Alternatively, dobutamine stress echocardiography may be more specific for a finding of ischemia and is generally less costly.[8,9]

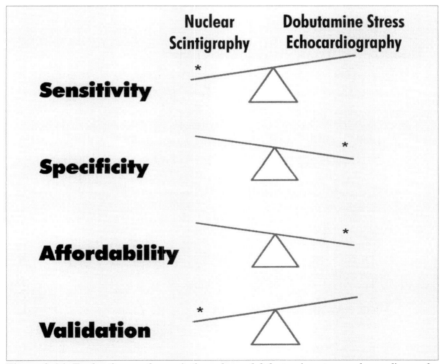

Figure 9-16. *Evaluating nuclear scintigraphy and dobutamine stress echocardiography to detect myocardial ischemia.*

PATIENTS WITHOUT HISTORY OF ANGINA OR MYOCARDIAL INFARCTION

The likelihood of coronary disease in heart failure patients without angina or history of MI varies with patient risk factors for coronary artery disease. Although practice varies, consider screening patients for myocardial ischemia who have heart failure and significant risk factors for atherosclerosis (e.g., age, sex, smoking history, hyperlipidemia, hypertension, family history of premature coronary artery disease, and diabetes).

Chronic Pressure or Volume Overload
Systolic Dysfunction

Chronic pressure overload due to hypertension or aortic stenosis commonly leads to concentric hypertrophy of the left ventricle with a decrease in left ventricular internal chamber dimension and a decrease in left ventricular diastolic compliance. Systolic function is preserved. If pressure overload is sustained, however, dilated hypertrophy may gradually develop and result in systolic dysfunction heart failure.

Initially, left ventricular volume overload leads to an *increase* in left ventricular ejection fraction. *Over time*, however, progressive dilatation of the left ventricle is associated with a progressive *decrease* in ejection fraction. Forward stroke volume is relatively preserved. Ultimately, a dilated left ventricle with poor systolic function results.

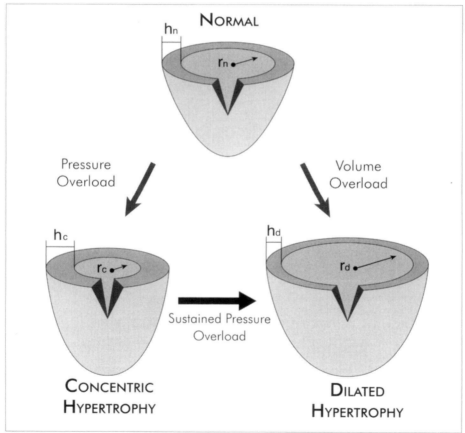

Figure 9-17. *Chronic pressure overload leads to concentric hypertrophy in which the radius decreases and the wall thickness increases. Sustained volume overload results in dilated hypertrophy in which the radius increases and the wall thickness decreases from normal.*

Dilated Cardiomyopathy

PRIMARY CAUSES OF MYOCARDIAL DYSFUNCTION

Unfortunately, the majority of patients with dilated non-ischemic cardiomyopathy due to primary myocardial disease have no identifiable cause for their heart failure. If you can identify an etiology, however, specific treatment can often improve outcome.[10] Familial dilated cardiomyopathy implies a genetic etiology of ventricular dysfunction and accounts for up to 35% of patients with "idiopathic" dilated cardiomyopathy.[11] To date, only a small number of specific genetic causes of familial cardiomyopathy have been identified.[12-14] Many more are likely to be found in the future.

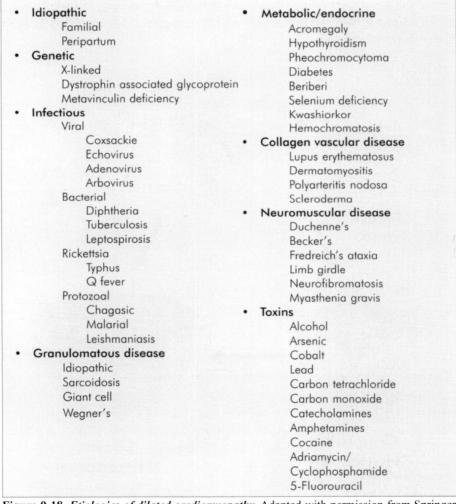

- **Idiopathic**
    - Familial
    - Peripartum
- **Genetic**
    - X-linked
    - Dystrophin associated glycoprotein
    - Metavinculin deficiency
- **Infectious**
    - Viral
        - Coxsackie
        - Echovirus
        - Adenovirus
        - Arbovirus
    - Bacterial
        - Diphtheria
        - Tuberculosis
        - Leptospirosis
    - Rickettsia
        - Typhus
        - Q fever
    - Protozoal
        - Chagasic
        - Malarial
        - Leishmaniasis
- **Granulomatous disease**
    - Idiopathic
    - Sarcoidosis
    - Giant cell
    - Wegner's

- **Metabolic/endocrine**
    - Acromegaly
    - Hypothyroidism
    - Pheochromocytoma
    - Diabetes
    - Beriberi
    - Selenium deficiency
    - Kwashiorkor
    - Hemochromatosis
- **Collagen vascular disease**
    - Lupus erythematosus
    - Dermatomyositis
    - Polyarteritis nodosa
    - Scleroderma
- **Neuromuscular disease**
    - Duchenne's
    - Becker's
    - Fredreich's ataxia
    - Limb girdle
    - Neurofibromatosis
    - Myasthenia gravis
- **Toxins**
    - Alcohol
    - Arsenic
    - Cobalt
    - Lead
    - Carbon tetrachloride
    - Carbon monoxide
    - Catecholamines
    - Amphetamines
    - Cocaine
    - Adriamycin/ Cyclophosphamide
    - 5-Fluorouracil

Figure 9-18. *Etiologies of dilated cardiomyopathy.* Adapted with permission from Springer-Verlag. Hosenpud JD. The cardiomyopathies. In: Congestive heart failure: Pathophysiology, diagnosis, and comprehensive approach to management. 1994:199.[10]

DILATED CARDIOMYOPATHY (IDIOPATHIC/OTHER) IN LAB TESTING

The lab tests to the right can screen patients with dilated cardiomyopathy to rule out treatable secondary etiologies.[15] Obtaining an iron (Fe^{++}) and iron binding capacity (TIBC) provides an index for cardiomyopathy related to iron overload; either hemochromatosis or secondary iron overload due to multiple transfusions or ineffective bone marrow erythropoiesis. An

LAB TESTS
• Fe^{++}/TIBC or Ferritin
• Thyroid Panel
If Clinically Indicated:
• Antinuclear Antibodies
• ESR

elevated iron–iron binding capacity ratio of greater than 50% and a ferritin level greater than 200 µg per liter are consistent with this diagnosis. In women with iron overload cardiomyopathy, these levels may be lower.

Recently the etiology of hereditary hemochromatosis has been related to an iron loading gene on human chromosome six associated with a recessive pattern of inheritance.[16] This gene occurs in as many as 10% of subjects of European origin who are clinically unaffected heterozygotes. Three to five per 1000 are homozygotes with a potentially lethal iron overload involving the heart, liver, pancreas, joints, and endocrine glands.

The heart may be involved with either a dilated or restrictive type cardiomyopathy by echocardiography. The dilated cardiomyopathy may be a more advanced stage of the disorder. In either case, confirmation of the diagnosis can be made by a characteristic reduced signal by magnetic resonance imaging or by endomyocardial biopsy showing increased iron stores within myocytes. Electron microscopy will show marked electron dense bodies within myocytes. Chelation therapy (intravenous deferoxamine) may lead to reversal of findings of heart failure due to cardiac iron overload.[16]

☑ *Chelation therapy with deferoxamine may reverse systolic or diastolic dysfunction due to iron overload.*

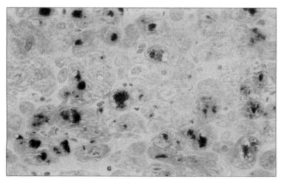

Figure 9-19. *This slide of an endomyocardial biopsy (prepared with Prussian blue stain) shows increased iron deposits within the myocytes of a patient with hemochromatosis.*

Either hyper- or hypo-thyroidism may lead to heart failure. Hyperthyroidism can present with high output heart failure with or without atrial fibrillation — both should respond to treatment of hyperthyroidism with propothyoruracil, radioactive iodine or β-blockers. Hypothyroidism can produce dilated cardiomyopathy. This may relate to changes in myosin gene expression mediated by the level of thyroid hormone. This should respond to thyroid replacement.

☑ *ESR in heart failure is usually low in the absence of inflammation.*

Anti-nuclear antibodies are a useful screen for inflammatory conditions including systemic lupus erythematosis. An erythrocyte sedimentation rate (ESR) is a non-specific screening for inflammatory conditions including viral or idiopathic myocarditis.

There is no specific treatment for myocarditis. In general, immunosuppression is not beneficial.[17] Biopsy proven myocarditis, however, can indicate a need to delay cardiac transplant, with mechanical support if necessary, since LV dysfunction may improve spontaneously.[18] Furthermore, heart transplants performed in patients with active biopsy proven myocarditis have a poor outcome with a decreased 58% one-year survival.[17]

☑ *Myocardial dysfunction due to myocarditis often improves spontaneously.*

In situations suggested by history of being in endemic regions, unusual causes of infections involving the heart such as Chagas' disease may be important to exclude. In patients who otherwise have "idiopathic dilated cardiomyopathy" after screening, it is not mandatory to perform endomyocardial biopsy.

Peripartum Cardiomyopathy

Peripartum cardiomyopathy is a type of idiopathic dilated cardiomyopathy with clinical onset between the last month of pregnancy and the first six months postpartum. It is unknown if this presentation is due to a specific etiology related to pregnancy or an unmasking of left ventricular dysfunction of a preexisting cause.[19] Although the findings of heart failure may regress within six months of symptom onset,[20] peripartum cardiomyopathy may also lead to either death or need for heart transplant. The incidence in a large series was 28 out of 67,369 deliveries (4/10,000).[19] Clinical suspicion is necessary to obtain an echocardiogram which leads to the diagnosis.

☑ *Peripartum cardiomyopathy may present from the last month of pregnancy until six months postpartum.*

Cardiomyopathy due to Sustained Supraventricular Tachycardia

Dilated cardiomyopathy may occur secondary to a sustained supraventricular tachycardia. The abnormal rhythm may be atrial fibrillation, reentrant, or ectopic atrial tachycardia. Ablation of the tachycardia may lead to total resolution of the left ventricular dysfunction.[21]

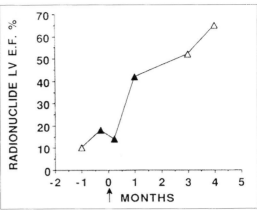

Figure 9-20. *Increases in left ventricular ejection fraction versus time following ablation of an ectopic atrial tachycardia in a patient with non-ischemic cardiomyopathy.* Reprinted with permission from Mosby, Inc. Rabbani LE, et al. Time course of improvement in ventricular function after ablation of incessant automatic atrial tachycardia. Am.Heart J. 1991; 121:819.[21]

Transvenous Cardiac Biopsy: Endomyocardial Biopsy (EMB)

Percutaneous transvenous myocardial biopsy performed from the right internal jugular vein remains the test of choice for diagnosis of cardiac transplant rejection and for assessment of adriamycin cardiotoxicity. In addition, endomyocardial biopsy is useful for the diagnosis of hemochromatosis, primary amyloidosis, or sarcoidosis. When identified, these conditions offer potential specific treatment. When EMB identifies a histologic type of cardiomyopathy, open-thoracotomy attempt at pericardial stripping

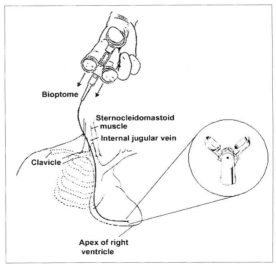

Figure 9-21. *Myocardial biopsy technique.*

to exclude constrictive pericarditis may be avoided. Rare findings of EMB include Loffler's endomyocardial fibrosis, Fabry's disease, and the glycogen storage diseases.[22]

Diastolic Dysfunction

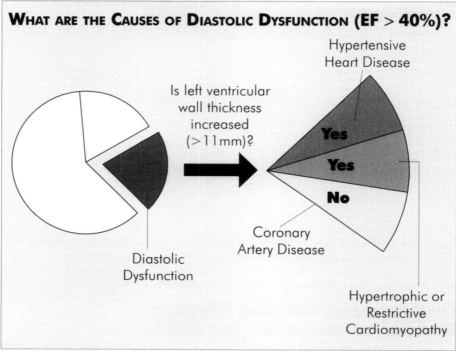

Figure 9-22. *Causes of diastolic dysfunction and associated left ventricular wall thickness.*

You can make the diagnosis of diastolic dysfunction heart failure when clinical findings of lung congestion, often by chest x-ray, are found with a preserved systolic function of the left ventricle — ejection fraction greater than 40%. Diastolic dysfunction is often associated with left ventricular hypertrophy indicated by a wall thickness greater than 11 mm by echocardiography. When left ventricular hypertrophy is not present by echocardiography, transient diastolic dysfunction may be present associated with coronary artery disease and acute myocardial ischemia.

☑ *Consider non-cardiac etiologies of interstitial infiltrates on chest x-ray when EF > 40%.*

Interstitial lung disease or non-cardiogenic pulmonary edema can mimic the findings of diastolic dysfunction since both are also associated with infiltrates on chest x-ray and preserved systolic function by echo. Interstitial lung disease does not improve with diuretics. Non-cardiogenic pulmonary edema (also called adult respiratory distress syndrome) is usually present in the patient who has an acute non-cardiac systemic illness. Despite these differences, you may have to measure a high pulmonary capillary wedge pressure by Swan-Ganz catheterization to confirm the presence of pulmonary infiltrates due to heart failure.

HYPERTENSIVE HEART DISEASE

Look for uniform hypertrophy and contraction of the ventricle.

When a patient, especially if elderly, with clinical heart failure has left ventricular hypertrophy by echo and a history of high blood pressure, the diagnosis of hypertensive heart disease is likely. The presence of other echo-Doppler findings of diastolic dysfunction (see below) help support this diagnosis. You should

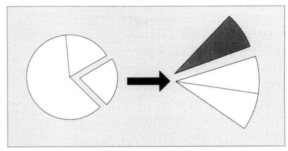

Figure 9-23. *A proportion of diastolic dysfunction is attributed to hypertensive heart disease.*

consider that patients with hypertensive heart disease may also have associated coronary artery disease. Significant ventricular hypertrophy *in the absence* of a history of high blood pressure often implies the presence of a secondary process due to either hypertrophic cardiomyopathy, infiltrative cardiomyopathy, or restrictive cardiomyopathy that may be associated with systemic illness.

ECHO-DOPPLER FINDINGS IN DIASTOLIC DYSFUNCTION

- Left ventricular hypertrophy (wall thickness >11 mm)
- Left atrial enlargement
- Mitral and pulmonary vein Doppler flow abnormalities
- Increased pulmonary artery systolic pressure estimated from velocity of tricuspid regurgitation

☑ *The most common causes of diastolic dysfunction are hypertension and coronary artery disease.*

HYPERTROPHIC OR RESTRICTIVE CARDIOMYOPATHY

Look for regional variations in wall thickness.

Hypertrophic and restrictive cardiomyopathies are associated with diastolic dysfunction. Hypertrophic cardiomyopathy can be defined as left and/or right ventricular hypertrophy occurring usually in an asymmetric pattern and often involving the interventricular septum not secondary to systemic hypertension.[2] Left ventricular

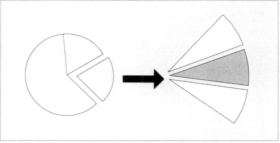

Figure 9-24. *A proportion of diastolic dysfunction is attributed to hypertrophic or restrictive overload.*

volume is normal or reduced. Microscopically, there is myocyte hypertrophy and disarray surrounding areas of increased loose connective tissue. It is often related to a genetic mutation in a sarcomere contractile protein (see pages 95–96). When hypertrophic cardiomyopathy is associated with left ventricular outflow gradient (idiopathic hypertrophic subaortic stenosis), management directed toward improving this gradient may be important. End-stage hypertrophic cardiomyopathy may progress to systolic dysfunction.

Restrictive cardiomyopathy can be defined as a condition of restricted ventricular filling and decreased ventricular volume with preserved systolic function. Amyloidosis, iron overload conditions, and idiopathic hypereosinophilia are potential causes of infiltrative or restrictive cardiomyopathy. Look for an associated systemic illness. Although left ventricular wall thickness can be normal, it is often increased due to infiltration of the interstitial space or intracellular volume of myocytes.[2]

CORONARY ARTERY DISEASE

Look for regional wall motion abnormalities.

As in patients with systolic dysfunction, regional wall motion abnormalities may indicate the presence of associated coronary artery disease. Usually, patients also have symptoms of angina. Screening for coronary artery disease is similar to that for patients with systolic dysfunction.

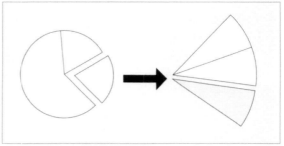

Figure 9-25. *A proportion of diastolic dysfunction is attributed to coronary artery disease.*

Doppler Flow Patterns Seen in Presence of Impaired Diastolic Dysfunction

Doppler echocardiography measures blood flow velocity versus time within the chambers of the heart. You can identify abnormalities of diastolic function by measuring blood flow velocities during diastole at the level of the mitral valve and within the pulmonary veins. Small left atrium to left ventricle (A, mitral flow) and pulmonary venous to left atrium (B, pulmonary venous flow) pressure gradients determine blood flow velocities.[23]

☑ *Doppler has been referred to as the "Rosetta Stone" of diastolic dysfunction.*[23]

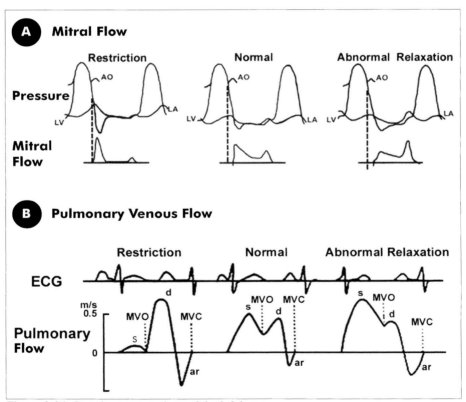

Figure 9-26. *Doppler presentations of the left heart.*

☑ *"E-A reversal" is the mitral flow pattern of abnormal relaxation.*

Normal mitral flow velocity consists of an early diastolic peak in filling followed by a smaller peak in filling following atrial contraction. At least two patterns of abnormalities of diastolic filling occur. Abnormal left ventricular relaxation is characterized by a decrease in early filling and a compensatory increase filling following atrial contraction leading to "E-A reversal" of normal velocity ratios. Alternatively, a restrictive filling pattern is characterized by a markedly increased left atrial pressure during rapid early filling and an increase in the ratio of E to A peak velocities.

☑ *Changes in LV preload can affect Doppler diastolic flow patterns.*

Pulmonary venous flow velocity signals are technically more difficult to obtain. Normal systolic flow (s) into the left atrium of the pulmonary veins exceeds diastolic flow (d). Atrial contraction leads to a reversal of flow (ar) from the left atrium to the pulmonary veins (Figure 9-26). Pulmonary venous flow velocity of diastolic dysfunction due to abnormal left ventricular relaxation is associated with a decrease in velocity during early diastolic filling. Subsequent *systolic* flow into the left atrium is *increased*. With restrictive left ventricular dysfunction and high left atrial pressure, systolic flow into the left atrium decreases, and flow into the left atrium is dependent on the emptying of the left atrium into the left ventricle during *early diastole*. Atrial reversal of flow after atrial contraction is also increased. Although myocardial diastolic relaxation and restriction abnormalities can coexist, it is useful to characterize which of these two Doppler patterns predominate.

Color M-mode and tissue Doppler are evolving techniques to study diastolic function. These methods may allow an estimate of LV relaxation that is relatively insensitive to the effects of changes in ventricular preload.[24]

Hypothesis

Diastolic dysfunction progresses from abnormal relaxation to restrictive impaired diastolic compliance.[12]

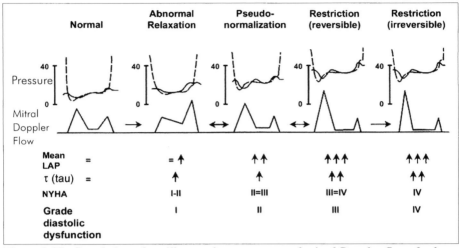

Figure 9-27. *Correlation of capillary wedge pressures and mitral Doppler flows for heart failure.* Reprinted with permission from the American College of Cardiology (Journal of the American College of Cardiology, July 1997; 30:13).[23]

Isolated diastolic dysfunction of the left ventricle is clinically manifest as an increase in left atrial or pulmonary capillary wedge pressure despite a normal or reduced left ventricular chamber size. In a research catheterization lab environment, left ventricular isovolumic relaxation or pressure decrease within the left ventricle following aortic valve closure can be characterized by the exponential time constant τ (tau) (see page 54).

Worsening diastolic dysfunction with increasing left atrial pressure (LAP) may be associated with a progression of diastolic mitral flow velocity abnormalities. Doppler flow may progress from normal to abnormal relaxation to restriction. Between abnormal relaxation and restriction, a Doppler flow pattern similar to normal occurs called pseudo-normalization. It can be difficult to distinguish normal from pseudo-normalization pattern based on the mitral flow velocity profile alone. A Valsalva maneuver can change the pseudo-normalization pattern to an abnormal relaxation pattern with E-A reversal. Conversely, a Valsalva maneuver with a normal flow velocity reduces both E and A velocity without E-A reversal.

☑ *A Valsalva maneuver can help distinguish a normal versus pseudo-normal Doppler flow pattern.*

Diastolic Dysfunction due to Hypertrophic Cardiomyopathy

TYPES OF HYPERTROPHIC CARDIOMYOPATHY

- Idiopathic Hypertrophic Subaortic Stenosis (IHSS)
    or Hypertrophic Obstructive Cardiomyopathy (HOCM)
- Apical Hypertrophy
- Symmetric Hypertrophy

Patients with hypertrophic cardiomyopathy represent a small but important subset within the spectrum of patients with heart failure because treatment differs significantly from treatment of other causes. Hypertrophic cardiomyopathy can arise from either an inherited or a spontaneous mutation in a gene coding for a protein within the sarcomere, most commonly the heavy chain of myosin. The prevalence of all forms of hypertrophic cardiomyopathy may be as common as one in 500 in the United States population; however, many patients are asymptomatic.[25]

The pattern of hypertrophy within the left (or right) ventricle between individuals can vary, even within a single family. All share the common functional feature of diastolic dysfunction. Echocardiography visualizes the distribution of hypertrophy.

☑ *Routine genetic identification of a patient with suspected hypertrophic cardiomyopathy is not available at present but may be in the future.*

The most common pattern is asymmetric septal hypertrophy with a ratio of septal to posterior wall thickness of 1.3 or greater. In the United States, idiopathic hypertrophic subaortic stenosis (IHSS) is the name of this type of hypertrophic cardiomyopathy (Figure 9-28). This is usually accompanied by findings of dynamic left ventricular outflow tract obstruction with a systolic murmur that can simulate aortic valve stenosis. When present, there is typically systolic anterior motion of the mitral valve and an increase in Doppler velocity across the left ventricular outflow tract during systolic ejection. A characteristic "spike and dome" morphology may be found in the aortic pressure or left ventricular outflow tract velocity with dynamic outflow tract obstruction. This pattern arises from an initial unobstructed ejection of blood from the left ventricle followed by progressive obstruction of outflow during the period of mid-to-late systolic ejection.

Figure 9-28. *IHSS – idio-pathic hypertrophic subaortic stenosis characterized by a ratio of septal to posterior wall thickness of 1.3 or greater.*

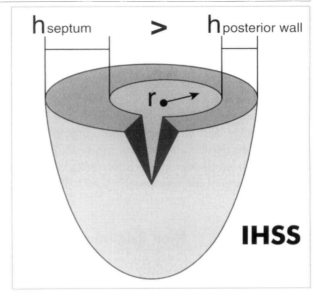

☑ *You should distinguish LV outflow tract obstruction due to IHSS from valvular aortic stenosis.*

In IHSS, medications such as digoxin or catecholamines that increase myo-cardial contractility will increase dynamic left ventricular outflow tract obstruc-tion and potentially worsen the findings of heart failure. Excessive vasodilation can worsen left ventricular outflow gradient and pump function. Excessive di-uresis can reduce left ventricular size and also increase functional outflow tract gradient.

Conversely, β-blockers that decrease contractility will lead to hemodynamic improvement in IHSS by decreasing outflow tract obstruction (as opposed to the delayed improvement of β-blockers in dilated cardiomyopathy). The calcium channel blocker, verapamil, with negative inotropic and bradycardic effects may also improve left ventricular outflow obstruction but must be used cautiously since its action as an arteriolar vasodilator tends to produce the opposite effect.

A less common manifestation of hypertrophic cardiomyopathy is hypertro-phy confined to the apex of the left ventricle. This pattern can occur associated with marked T-wave inversion across the precordial leads on a standard 12-lead electrocardiogram.

Diffuse concentric hypertrophy of the left ventricle may be another type of hypertrophic cardiomyopathy. This is the same pattern of hypertrophy seen sec-ondary to hypertension or infiltrative causes of cardiomyopathy. In the absence of history of hypertension or family history of hypertrophic cardiomyopathy, con-sider performing an endomyocardial biopsy to exclude alternative diagnoses in these cases.

Counsel patients after making the diagnosis of hypertrophic cardiomyopathy. Especially in the young individual, with or without symptoms, a patient can become severely depressed because of the potential chronic and progressive nature of the disorder. It is important to emphasize that many patients have a benign prognosis with an annual mortality in unselected populations of 1% or less.[26] Screen immediate family members for hypertrophic cardiomyopathy with echocardiography. In patients with significant left ventricular outflow tract obstruction (> 50 mm Hg), patients should avoid vigorous levels of exercise since sudden death with exertion may be an initial manifestation of the problem. On the other hand, reassure adults with hypertrophic cardiomyopathy if they have none of the following high risk indicators.[26]

HIGH RISK INDICATORS IN IHSS

- Symptoms with activity
- Family history of premature death
- Nonsustained ventricular tachycardia during ambulatory electrocardiographic monitoring
- Marked outflow tract gradient (> 50 mm Hg)
- Substantial left ventricular hypertrophy more than 20 mm
- Marked left atrial enlargement
- Abnormal blood pressure fall with exercise

Diastolic Dysfunction due to Restrictive Cardiomyopathy

Causes of diastolic dysfunction other than hypertension, coronary artery disease, or hypertrophic cardiomyopathy are numerous but less common. When a diagnosis of idiopathic restrictive cardiomyopathy is made, it is usually done in the setting of objective findings of congestion either by chest x-ray or by direct measurement of elevated pulmonary capillary wedge pressure. At this point it is also important to exclude the possible treatable finding of constrictive pericarditis. Unfortunately, specific treatment is unavailable for most restrictive cardiomyopathy. Although wall thickness is usually increased, it may be normal.

DIASTOLIC DYSFUNCTION DUE TO RESTRICTIVE CARDIOMYOPATHY (LVEF > 40)

MYOCARDIAL
- **INFILTRATIVE**
  Amyloidosis
  Sarcoidosis
  Gaucher's disease
  Hurler's disease
  Fatty infiltration

- **NONINFILTRATIVE**
  Hypertrophic cardiomyopathy
  Idiopathic cardiomyopathy
  Familial cardiomyopathy
  Scleroderma
  Pseudoxanthoma elasticum
  Diabetic cardiomyopathy
  Hemochromatosis

- **STORAGE DISEASES**
  Fabry's disease
  Glycogen storage disease

ENDOMYOCARDIAL
Endomyocardial fibrosis
Idiopathic fibrosis
Hypereosinophilic syndrome
Carcinoid heart disease
Metastatic cancer
Radiation
Toxic effects of adriamycin
Drugs causing fibrous endocarditis
(serotonin, methysergide, ergotamine, mercurial agents, busulfan)

Figure 9-29. *Classification of types of restrictive cardiomyopathy according to cause.* Reprinted with permission from The New England Journal of Medicine, copyright © 1997 Massachusetts Medical Society. All rights reserved. (New England Journal of Medicine, 1997; 336:268).[27]

☑ *Hemochromatosis may result in either a restrictive or dilated cardiomyopathy.*

Restrictive Cardiomyopathy due to Amyloidosis

The most common identifiable cause of restrictive cardiomyopathy is amyloidosis, either primary including that associated with multiple myeloma or secondary associated with chronic inflammation.[14] By echocardiography, the left and right ventricles are both hypertrophied usually with a "speckled" visual appearance within the thickened walls. Systolic function is usually preserved, but not hyperdynamic as it may be with hypertensive or hypertrophic cardiomyopathy. Diagnosis is supported by findings of associated immunoglobulin on serum protein electrophoresis or confirmed by endomyocardial biopsy showing interstitial myocardial deposition of amyloid protein. Prognosis with amyloidosis restrictive cardiomyopathy is worse than with primary restrictive cardiomyopathy.[10] At present, no disease specific treatment exists for amyloidosis-related cardiomyopathy, although potential therapies are in evaluation.[28] Following cardiac transplantation, amyloid deposits will recur in the transplanted heart.[29]

☑ *Amyloidosis is the most common identifiable cause of restrictive cardiomyopathy.*

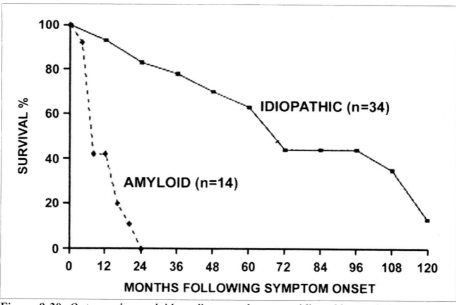

Figure 9-30. *Outcome in amyloid cardiomyopathy versus idiopathic restrictive cardiomyopathy.* Reprinted with permission from Springer-Verlag. Hosenpud JD. The cardiomyopathies. In: Congestive heart failure: Pathophysiology, diagnosis, and comprehensive approach to mangement.1994:205.[10]

Three Potentially Treatable Diagnoses Other Than Systolic or Diastolic Dysfunction

An echocardiogram can reveal three potentially treatable diagnoses other than systolic or diastolic heart failure. These conditions require treatment distinct from left ventricular dyfunction. Any may be a sole diagnosis or a new precipitant for deterioration in a patient with previously compensated heart failure.

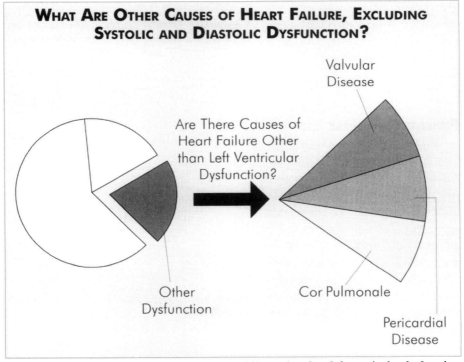

Figure 9-31. *Potentially treatable causes of heart failure other than left ventricular dysfunction.*

VALVULAR DISEASE

Valvular heart disease can lead to heart failure due to left ventricular volume overload: aortic or mitral regurgitation; or pressure overload: aortic stenosis; or restricted left ventricular filling: mitral stenosis. Color Doppler and derived formulae can quantitate the severity of the anatomically visualized lesion in all of these cases. Valve replacement or repair can often reverse findings of heart failure.

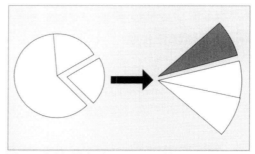

Figure 9-32. *Valvular causes of heart failure can often be reversed with valve replacement or repair.*

PERICARDIAL DISEASE

Pericardial disease may simulate left or right heart failure. Elevation of pericardial pressure will simulate ventricular diastolic dysfunction and will be associated with a parallel shift upward in the left and right ventricular diastolic pressure-volume curve (see page 65). Major types of pericardial disease include pericardial effusion with tamponade and pericardial constriction.

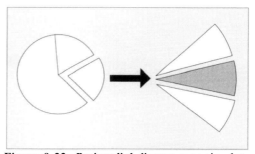

Figure 9-33. *Pericardial disease may simulate heart failure.*

COR PULMONALE

Cor Pulmonale is defined as right sided heart failure secondary to pulmonary disease associated with high pulmonary artery pressure. If you can treat and improve the reason for excessive right ventricular afterload, right heart failure can improve.

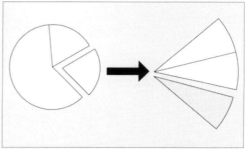

Figure 9-34. *Treating Cor Pulmonale may improve the status of right heart failure.*

Valvular Heart Disease

Valvular heart disease represents an important treatable cause of heart failure. Valvular heart disease may be acquired or congenital. In the adult, the major types of valvular disease associated with heart failure are mechanical deformities of the aortic or mitral valve. When valvular disease is responsible for clinical heart failure, consider surgical correction. In the adult, congenital heart disease is a less common cause of either pressure or volume overload of either ventricle.

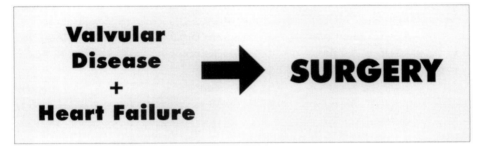

Aortic Stenosis

The typical murmur of aortic stenosis is a systolic ejection murmur best heard along the left and right upper sternal border radiating to the carotid arteries. In patients with aortic stenosis and heart failure, the murmur may be difficult to auscultate due to low heart output. In patients in cardiogenic shock, echocardiography may be the only way to identify aortic stenosis.

By echo, the aortic valve appears calcified and restricted in motion. The pressure gradient across the valve can be estimated by the Bernoulli equation as $\Delta P = 4\ v_{Ao}^2$ where v_{Ao} is the peak velocity across the valve by continuous

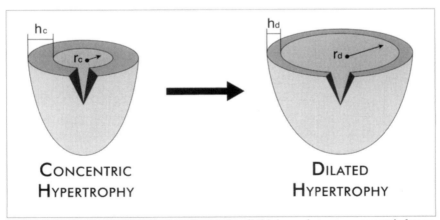

Figure 9-35. *Notice the change in radius and wall thickness between concentric hypertrophy and dilated hypertrophy.*

wave Doppler interrogation. The valve area can be assessed by the continuity equation that incudes measurement at the left ventricle outflow tract, LVOT, by the equation $Area_{Ao} = (v_{LVOT}/v_{Ao}) \times Area_{LVOT}$.

VARIABLES
V_{AO} — peak velocity across valve by Doppler
LVOT — left ventricular outflow tract
V_{LVOT} — Doppler velocity at LVOT
$Area_{LVOT}$ — cross-sectional area of LVOT by 2 dimensional echocardiography

Cardiac catheterization directly measures the valve pressure gradient and, with a thermodilution or Fick cardiac output, yields a calculated valve area.

A pressure gradient greater than or equal to 50 mm Hg or valve area less than or equal to 0.7 cm^2 usually indicates hemodynamically significant aortic stenosis.[30]

If a patient has heart failure and aortic stenosis, a small valve area may be present associated with only a moderate pressure gradient. If aortic valve area is reduced and there is a low ejection fraction, you should consider aortic valve replacement surgery if the mean valve gradient is greater than or equal to 30 mm Hg.[31]

AORTIC REGURGITATION

Left ventricular volume overload due to aortic regurgitation can be acute or chronic.[32] Acute aortic regurgitation with a non-dilated left ventricle is often associated with bacterial endocarditis of the aortic valve or aortic root dissection. Chronic aortic regurgitation may be due to aortic root dilatation or congenitally deformed bicuspid aortic valve. Marfan's Syndrome, rheumatic heart disease, and rheumatoid arthritis are also associated with aortic regurgitation. Chronic severe aortic regurgitation can lead to dramatic physical exam findings including wide pulse pressure, visibly bounding, double (or bisfiriens) pulse, and marked cardiomegaly. When heart failure

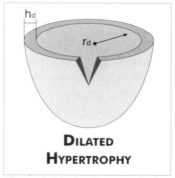

DILATED HYPERTROPHY

Figure 9-36. *Aortic regurgitation results in dilated hypertrophy.*

is present, aortic valve surgery should be considered. Prognosis for aortic valve replacement is related to the degree of left ventricle chamber enlargement. In the absence of symptoms, progressive or marked left ventricular enlargement should also suggest a need for aortic valve replacement since an end-systolic dimension greater than 5.5 cm by echocardiography is associated with a poorer survival after surgery.[32]

☑ *Long-standing significant aortic regurgitation can lead to dramatic findings on physical exam.*

MITRAL REGURGITATION

Acute severe mitral regurgitation can cause pulmonary edema with a normal sized left ventricle and hyperdynamic left ventricular systolic function. Examples of this include bacterial mitral valve endocarditis or papillary muscle rupture associated with myocardial infarction, or chordae tendinae rupture associated with redundant mitral valve leaflets.

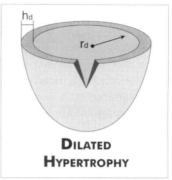

DILATED HYPERTROPHY

Figure 9-37. *Mitral regurgitation results in dilated hypertrophy.*

When *chronic* mitral regurgitation leads to heart failure it is usually with dilated hypertrophy of the left ventricle. Ultimately the dilated left ventricle fails due to excessive wall stress. When mitral regurgitation presents with a reduced left ventricular ejection fraction, it can be a challenge to determine if heart failure is secondary to mitral regurgitation or if mitral regurgitation is secondary to *other* causes of ventricular enlargement. Primary mitral regurgitation can be the result of rheumatic heart disease, mitral valve prolapse or mitral annular calcification. When mitral regurgitation is the cause for heart failure, either transthoracic or transesophageal echocardiography can identify mitral valve deformities suitable for mitral valve repair. If repair is not possible, preservation of the posterior valve apparatus can blunt subsequent ventricular enlargement associated with mitral valve replacement.

It is common for left ventricular ejection fraction to initially *decrease* after correction of mitral regurgitation because of elimination of ventricular systolic ejection retrograde into the low pressure left atrium.

MITRAL STENOSIS

Mitral stenosis usually develops decades after acute rheumatic fever. In the elderly, it can occur with calcification of the mitral annulus without previous rheumatic fever.[33] Patients typically present with symptoms of shortness of breath due to pulmonary congestion. Since the left ventricle is "protected" by the narrowed mitral valve, valve repair or replacement is usually associated with an excellent recovery of circulatory function. In patients with long-standing mitral stenosis associated with severe pulmonary hypertension, right ventricular failure manifested by symptoms of fatigue associated with a low cardiac output can predomi-

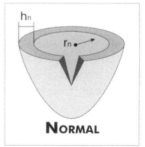

NORMAL

Figure 9-38. *Mitral stenosis maintains a normal radius and thickness.*

nate. The increase in resistance to flow through the pulmonary arterial circulation is known as the "second stenosis" in patients with mitral stenosis. Operative risk is higher and functional recovery impaired when high pulmonary vascular resistance is associated with right ventricular failure preoperatively.

VALVE REPLACEMENT OR REPAIR

Surgical valve replacement or repair remains the treatment of choice for heart failure secondary to significant aortic or mitral valve disease. In chronic valve dysfunction, the most dramatic results are obtained with aortic stenosis or mitral stenosis. Typically intrinsic left ventricular dysfunction is more profound in volume overload mitral regurgitation or aortic regurgitation when these lesions have culminated in symptoms of heart failure.[33]

When atrial fibrillation is present preoperatively, concomitant surgical treatment of the atria via a Maze procedure may provide a better hemodynamic result if sinus rhythm can be sustained.[34]

PERCUTANEOUS MITRAL VALVULOPLASTY

Percutaneous mitral valvuloplasty using balloon catheters to dilate a stenotic mitral valve can be considered an alternative to open valve repair or replacement in appropriate patients. In a meta-analysis series[30] on average, mitral valve area increased from 1.0 to 2.0 cm^2 with reduction of mean valve gradient from 15 to 6 mm Hg. Mortality from this procedure was 0.5%. Other complications include cardiac perforation, pericardial tamponade, severe mitral regurgitation or cerebral vascular accident. In general, patients who have severely calcified valves will require open heart surgery to achieve a good result.[35] In patients with mitral stenosis but pliable valves, percutaneous mitral valvuloplasty may be preferable to surgical commissurotomy since it achieves similar results without the liabilities of thoracotomy and cardiopulmonary bypass.[36]

Results from percutaneous balloon valvuloplasty in aortic stenosis, however, are much less beneficial with a high rate of recurrence.

CONGENITAL HEART DISEASE

A congenital heart lesion in an adult may be unrecognized or known. If previously diagnosed, the abnormality may have been either observed, palliated, or corrected. Diverse lesions can occur: left-right shunts; right-left shunts (cyanotic heart disease); stenosis or hypoplasia of heart valves or ventricles; or great vessel abnormalities. Echocardiography and transesophageal echocardiography are usually adequate to define the anatomic and functional significance of a suspected congenital lesion. Atrial or ventricular arrhythmias may occur associated with any significant congenital heart lesion even years after successful surgical correction.

Atrial septal defect with left-right shunting is the most common significant lesion to be discovered initially as an adult. This typically results in right ventricular volume overload findings associated with a pulmonic valve systolic murmur due to increased flow. If associated with symptoms or if a pulmonary-systemic flow ratio is greater than 1.5 to 1, then surgical patch closure should be considered. If patients are over 40 years old, coronary angiography to detect coronary artery disease should be performed prior to surgery. In general, consider consultation with a clinician experienced with adult congenital heart disease if echocardiography demonstrates a significant congenital abnormality.

Transesophageal Echocardiogram

Performance of trans-esophageal echo (TEE) is not mandatory in the diagnosis of valvular dysfunction and heart failure. Nevertheless, a transesophageal echo can be useful when questions remain after transthoracic echocardiography. Flail mitral valve leaflet due to chordal rupture, papillary muscle tear, or endocarditis often indicates a need for mitral valve surgery. TEE is also useful for better defini-tion of possible valvular

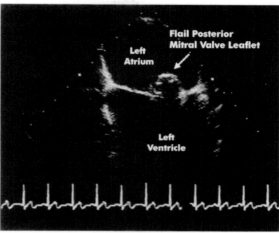

Figure 9-39. *Transesophageal echocardiogram demon-strating a flail posterior mitral valve leaflet.*

vegetations associated with endocarditis. TEE improves the assessment of pros-thetic tissue or mechanical valves, especially in the mitral position, since echogenic struts limit visualization with transthoracic echocardiography. Generally, the mitral valve is better assessed than the aortic valve given the close location of the left atrium to the esophagus.

Mechanical Valve Thrombosis

Although uncommon, patients with artificial mechanical valves can present with dramatic findings of decompensated heart failure due to valve thrombus formation despite long-term anticoagulation. Treatment options include surgi-cal repeat valve replacement and pharmacologic thrombolysis. Because of a 3-10% incidence of embolic cerebrovascular accident complications associ-ated with pharmacologic thrombolysis of obstructed left heart prosthetic valves, the treatment of choice in patients who are at low risk for surgical complications is early reoperation.[37]

Consider thrombolytic therapy for patients who are at high risk for reoperation valve surgery because of an advanced age or history of preexisting heart failure after transthoracic echocardiography or cinefluoroscopy identifies an immobile valve leaflet. In a large series, Roudaut[38] reported that intravenous thrombolytic therapy had a clinical success rate of 85% for prosthetic aortic valve thrombosis compared to 63% with mitral valve thrombosis. Transesophageal echocardiography, which provides only limited visualization of the aortic valve, is primarily useful for prosthetic mitral valve dysfunction. Due to its small size, thrombus is usually *not* visible by echocardiography in cases of mechanical valve thrombosis. The most common thrombolytic drug used is streptokinase,

250,000-U bolus given over 30 minutes followed by an infusion of 100,000 U/h for 24-72 hours.[39] Surgical replacement of an affected valve in high-risk surgery patients may still be necessary when valve thrombus is identified by echocardiography or in cases where there is no response to thrombolytic therapy as obstruction is probably due to pannus or tissue in-growth.

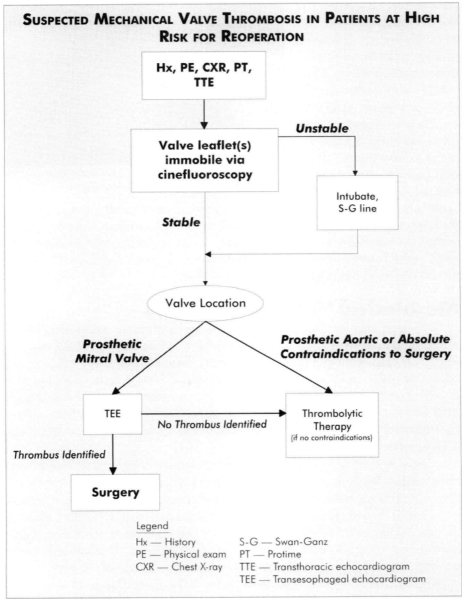

Figure 9-40. *Diagnostic and management algorithm of a suspected mitral or aortic mechanical valve thrombosis (St.Jude®, Carbomedics®, Bjork-Shiley®).*

Pericardial Disease

Rapid accumulation of fluid within the pericardium can cause acute pericardial tamponade with circulatory collapse with as little as 100 mL of pericardial fluid. Examples include postoperative open heart surgery bleeding, catheter related ventricular perforation, or post-myocardial infarction ventricular rupture. Intermediate diagnoses include effuso-constrictive disease that is usually confirmed when a significant pericardial effusion is drained and a residual elevation of ventricular filling pressures remains consistent with pericardial constriction. Neoplastic involvement of the pericardium commonly gives this finding and may be associated with a liter or more of effusion.

☑ *Rapidly increasing size of the cardiac silhouette on chest x-ray suggests a pericardial effusion.*

TYPES OF PERICARDIAL DISEASE

- Pericardial Tamponade
- Pericardial Constriction
- Effuso-constrictive Disease

FINDINGS OF TAMPONADE

- Pulsus paradox (> 10 mm Hg fall of blood pressure with inspiration)
- Hypotension
- Neck vein distention
- Electrical alternans on ECG
- Increase in size of cardiac silhouette on chest x-ray

ECHOCARDIOGRAPHIC FINDINGS OF TAMPONADE

- Large pericardial effusion (anterior and posterior to heart)
- RV collapse with inspiration
- RA collapse with inspiration
- Phasic changes in LVOT velocity

☑ *Pericardiocentesis in a patient with tamponade should lead to immediate improvement.*

Constrictive Pericarditis vs. Restrictive Cardiomyopathy

When a patient has heart failure despite normal left ventricular size and systolic function, distinguishing diastolic dysfunction due to restrictive cardiomyopathy from constrictive pericarditis can be an important clinical problem. Whereas pericardial stripping can lead to marked improvement with constrictive pericarditis, no surgical therapy will improve restrictive cardiomyopathy.[40]

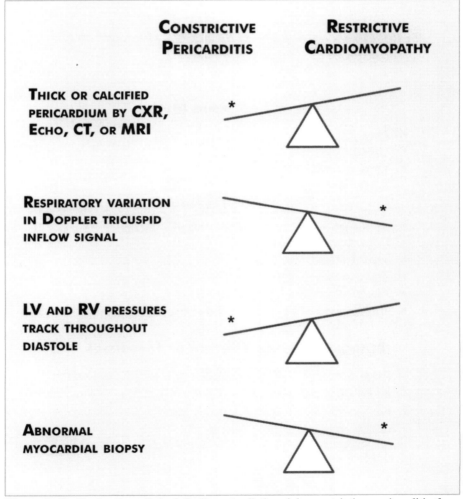

Figure 9-41. *Evaluating clinical findings to distinguish constrictive pericarditis from restrictive cardiomyopathy.*

A past medical history of acute pericarditis or tuberculosis favors constrictive pericarditis. Conversely, a systemic illness, such as amyloidosis, favors restrictive cardiomyopathy.

Physical findings can help distinguish the two conditions. A functionally rigid pericardium in constrictive pericarditis prevents respiratory variation of right ventricular filling. The constrictive pericardium becomes a rigid boot surrounding the heart. Typically, therefore, constrictive pericarditis — but not restrictive cardiomyopathy — occurs with a paradoxical increase in central venous pressure with respiration (positive Kussmaul sign). By Doppler echocardiography techniques, preservation of respiratory variation in tricuspid valve flow favors cardiomyopathy. In general, right and left filling pressures are markedly elevated with preserved systolic function in both conditions. Identical tracking of right and left ventricular diastolic pressure tracings prior to an "a" wave favors constriction. Abnormal histologic findings on endomyocardial biopsy favors restriction. Occasionally, pericardial constriction can *coexist* with restrictive cardiomyopathy such as following a previous episode of myopericarditis.[41] Final validation of constrictive pericarditis requires finding marked hemodynamic improvement following pericardial stripping.[40,42]

Marked right ventricular dysfunction with enlargement can simulate constrictive physiology, including an elevated intrapericardial pressure. This is important to differentiate from constrictive pericarditis since a pericardial stripping procedure will not benefit the patient with right ventricular failure. Medical therapy leading to improvement in right heart failure, however, will decrease left and right heart filling pressures through a reduction in intrapericardial pressure. This is a type of diastolic ventricular interaction due to pericardial constraint, septal transmission of pressure, and the effect of circumferential myocardial fibers that encircle both ventricular chambers.

☑ *Marked right ventricular enlargement can simulate pericardial constriction.*

Cor Pulmonale

Cor Pulmonale can present with findings of low cardiac output (fatigue or hypotension) and elevated right heart filling pressure (edema, ascites, and jugular venous distension). The echo in Cor Pulmonale reveals a large right ventricle, a small left ventricle, and a flattened intraventricular septum. Together this gives an appearance of a "D" sign on a short axis cross-section of the left ventricle as shown below.

Cor Pulmonale may occur secondary to either acute or chronic pulmonary emboli, chronic obstructive lung disease, or obesity related hypoventilation syndrome. Pulmonary hypertension due to left heart failure or congenital left to right shunts are not considered Cor Pulmonale. You can make the diagnosis of primary pulmonary hypertension in the presence of a high pulmonary vascular resistance of unknown cause after thorough evaluation to exclude secondary causes of pulmonary hypertension, especially pulmonary emboli. Recent trials have shown benefit with long-term intravenous prostacyclin therapy for primary pulmonary hypertension.[43]

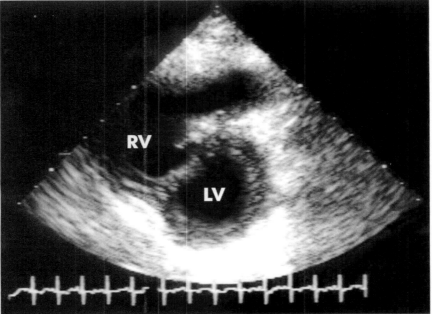

Figure 9-42. Echocardiographic LV "D" sign of right ventricular pressure overload.

☑ *Long-term intravenous prostacyclin therapy can improve prognosis in primary pulmonary hypertension.*

Chapter 9 Case Scenarios

SCENARIO #1

MEDICAL HISTORY
69-year-old female with 6-week history of increasing shortness of breath. History of hypertension. No history of angina or MI.

PHYSICAL EXAM
160/90 100 reg
Neck veins increased
Bibasilar rales
2/6 Systolic Ejection
Murmur (SEM) S_4
Trace edema

ECG
Increased QRS voltage
NS ST changes

CHEST X-RAY
Cardiomegaly
Increased interstitial pattern

ECHOCARDIOGRAM
Left ventricle: diffuse hypokinesis
EF < 20%
4 chamber enlargement

DOPPLER
Mild regurgitation

Question 1a

What test would you recommend for this patient next?

a) Adenosine ^{99m}Tc-sestamibi stress test

b) Swan-Ganz catheter

c) Cardiac catheterization

d) Endomyocardial biopsy

e) V/Q scan

f) none of the above

SCENARIO #1 CONTINUED

How would your recommendations change in Scenario #1 if the Echocardiogram and Doppler showed the following results?

1b)

ECHOCARDIOGRAM

LEFT VENTRICLE: Hyperdynamic EF
Asymmetric septal hypertrophy
Systolic anterior motion of the mitral valve

DOPPLER

Peak LVOT velocity 3 m/s
   (36 mm Hg)
Moderate mitral regurgitation

1c)

ECHOCARDIOGRAM

LEFT VENTRICLE: Hyperdynamic
EF = 80%
Concentric hypertrophy
End-systolic cavity obliteration
Aortic sclerosis

DOPPLER

E-A reversal

1d)

ECHOCARDIOGRAM

LEFT VENTRICLE: small chamber with
   flattened septum
EF = 60%
RIGHT VENTRICLE: Dilated, hypokinetic

DOPPLER

E-A reversal

1e)

ECHOCARDIOGRAM

LEFT VENTRICLE: Mild diffuse hypokinesis
EF = 50%
Concentric hypertrophy
Sclerocalcific changes aortic valve with
   decreased cusp separation

DOPPLER

Peak LVOT velocity 4.5 m/s
   (80 mm Hg)

LEGEND

LVOT — left ventricular outflow tract
EF — Ejection Fraction

SCENARIO #2

MEDICAL HISTORY
72-year-old male with a history of DM and abrupt onset of severe shortness of breath at 1 a.m.

CHEST X-RAY
Cardiomegaly
Infiltrates c/w pulmonary edema

PHYSICAL EXAM
160/90 100 reg
Neck veins increased
Bibasilar rales
S_4, 2/6 SEM
Trace edema

ECHOCARDIOGRAM
LEFT VENTRICLE: Normal
RIGHT VENTRICLE: Normal
Mild aortic valve sclerosis

ECG
Increased QRS voltage
NS ST changes

TROPONIN I
Within normal limits

Question 2

What would you recommend for this patient?

a) Adenosine ^{99m}Tc-sestamibi stress test

b) Swan-Ganz catheter tailored Rx

c) Cardiac catheterization

d) Endomyocardial biopsy

SCENARIO #3

MEDICAL HISTORY
62-year-old female with 6-week history
of increasing shortness of breath and
history of hypertension.

PHYSICAL EXAM
160/90 100 reg
Neck veins increased
Bibasilar rales
2/6 SEM S$_4$
Trace edema

ECHOCARDIOGRAM
LEFT VENTRICLE: Mild diffuse hypokinesis
EF = 50%
Concentric hypertrophy with speckled pattern
RIGHT VENTRICLE: free wall hypertrophy

URINALYSIS
3+ protein

ECG
Decreased QRS voltage
NS ST changes

CHEST X-RAY
Cardiomegaly
Increased interstitial pattern

Question 3

What would you recommend for this patient?

a) Outpatient milrinone/dobutamine

b) Swan-Ganz catheter tailored Rx

c) Coronary arteriogram

d) Arrange for home hospice

e) Endomyocardial biopsy

See Appendix for solutions.

Outpatient Therapy

Chapter 10

Once a patient has a diagnosis of heart failure including assessments of left ventricular function and etiology, it is important to tailor therapies that will improve a patient's quality of life and survival. Effective outpatient management can reduce the need for hospitalization and, in turn, save health care resources. This chapter serves as a guide to patient treatment and counseling, paying special attention to multicenter trials and pharmacologic treatments.

Objectives and Priorities in Therapy

SYMPTOM VERSUS DISEASE PROGRESSION THERAPY

Symptom Treatment of Decompensated Heart Failure
1. Diuretics — Decrease vascular volume
2. Digoxin — Increase contractility
3. Vasodilators — Decrease vascular tone

Disease Progression Treatment of Compensated Heart Failure
1. ACE Inhibitors — Decrease ventricular enlargement, vascular hypertrophy
2. β-Blockers — Reduce ventricular enlargement, ventricular arrhythmias

---

Figure 10-1. *Therapy for decompensated heart failure focuses on the treatment of hemodynamics to alleviate symptoms whereas outpatient treatment of compensated heart failure emphasizes neurohormonal status to control disease progression.*

DECOMPENSATED HEART FAILURE

Outpatient therapy objectives and priorities of heart failure historically evolved from the treatment of symptomatic decompensated heart failure in the inpatient setting — where the priority was improving hemodynamics to alleviate symptoms. Arrhythmias occurring in the hospital could usually be treated promptly and neurohormonal status was given secondary importance to improved hemodynamics.

☑ *Objectives and priorities differ between the treatment of decompensated and compensated heart failure.*

COMPENSATED HEART FAILURE

Improving hemodynamics can acutely relieve symptoms of congestion or inadequate perfusion, but will not necessarily improve prognosis if neurohormonal stimulation remains sustained at an inappropriately high level. In a small trial, patients with heart failure treated with the potent vasodilator, minoxidil, had improved symptoms and an initial increase in ejection fraction. Despite this, both long-term morbid events and mortality *were higher in the treated group* compared to placebo presumably due to unchecked neurohormonal activation associated with this potent direct vasodilator.[1]

As reviewed in Part I, *The Problem of Heart Failure*, blunting neurohormonal stimulation in compensated heart failure may be the most important factor affecting long-term outcome — since these factors mediate disease progression. In addition to improving symptoms by acting as vasodilators, ACE inhibitors reduce ventricular enlargement (captopril)[2] and progression to clinical heart failure (enalapril).[3] β-blockade complements ACE inhibition.

Ventricular arrhythmias are also important in the outpatient setting since they may result in sudden death. Sudden death can also occur for reasons other than ventricular tachyarrhythmias. Avoiding metabolic abnormalities and appropriate use of β-blockers, amiodarone, and automatic implantable cardioverter defibrillators can be effective (see pages 185-187 and 188–189).

COMPENSATED HEART FAILURE - REVERSE DISEASE PROGRESSION

OBJECTIVES

1. Improve quality of life
2. Reduce morbidity
3. Reduce mortality

PRIORITIES

1. Neurohormonal Status
2. Arrhythmias
3. Hemodynamics

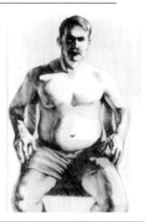

Figure 10-2. *Treatment of compensated heart failure.* Illustration by Peter Chapman.

Outpatient Counseling and Education

Patient education can include written materials to reinforce verbal instruction. Patients or their families should also know where to get additional information if desired. The Internet represents an increasingly accessible medium for obtaining information regarding all aspects of heart failure (for example, www.heartfailure.org).

Whenever possible, I recommend that patients walk on the level for 20-30 minutes one to two times per day. Some patients may benefit from a structured cardiac rehabilitation program with supervised exercise. During exercise, heart rate and blood pressure increase, however, following exercise heart rate and blood pressure decrease. This "hygienic approach" to neurohormonal withdrawal may contribute to the consistent benefit reported by studies of exercise rehabilitation in patients with heart failure.

> After you recognize that a patient has ventricular dysfunction, a patient should receive advice regarding the nature of heart failure, drug regimens, dietary restrictions, symptoms of worsening heart failure, what to do if symptoms occur, and prognosis.

Exercise may improve abnormalities of skeletal muscle physiology in patients with heart failure that can limit functional capacity.[4] Belardinelli and coworkers found that heart failure patients improved peak VO_2 by 18% two months after initiating a three times a week aerobic exercise training program at 60% baseline VO_2.[5] No change was seen in patients who did not exercise. Hare and coworkers found that patients who underwent resistance chest, shoulder, and knee exercise improved muscle strength and endurance. This type of exercise was not associated with an improvement in peak VO_2.[6]

Dietary instruction, when possible by a dietitian and/or heart failure clinician, is an integral part of treatment for patients with heart failure. Depending on the severity of heart failure, a patient should restrict his diet to 2-4 grams of sodium per day. A patient's total volume of fluid intake is a secondary concern unless a patient has a decreased serum sodium. In this case, a 1-2 liter fluid restriction should accompany a restriction of sodium intake. With heart failure due to coronary artery disease, patients should follow a diet that contributes to control of hyperlipidemia. If heart failure is advanced, patients may actually lose muscle weight (cardiac cachexia). They may feel too weak or short of breath to prepare and eat regular meals. If patients consistently lose weight, suggest a high calorie, high protein diet. Patients may also try eating smaller more frequent meals. Patients should measure and record weight at regular intervals.

Alcohol depresses myocardial function. In some individuals with "idiopathic cardiomyopathy," cessation of alcohol consumption leads to a marked improvement in myocardial function. In patients with mild to moderate left ventricular dysfunction, allowance of no more than one drink per day may offset the psychological burden imposed by other life style restrictions. In patients with a left ventricular ejection fraction of less than 30%, however, I recommend total abstinence of alcohol ingestion.[7]

Smoking cessation may be difficult for some patients. Nicotine patches, use of low doses of bupropion (Zyban®, Wellbutrin®) orally, or formal smoking cessation programs may help.[8]

Involvement of the patient's family in education and discussions of prognosis are important since lack of emotional support is a predictor of subsequent cardiovascular events.[9]

Activity	Recommendation
Exercise	Walking, cycling, etc. 20-30 minutes once to twice daily
Sodium intake	Restrict to close to 2 to 4 grams per day
Fluid Intake	In moderation, but less important than sodium intake
Calorie Intake	Appropriate to achieve ideal body weight
Alcohol consumption	Should be discouraged; patients who drink should be advised to consume no more than one drink per day (one drink equals a glass of beer or wine, or a mixed drink or cocktail containing no more than 1 ounce of alcohol)
Smoking	Immediate cessation

Figure 10-3. *Recommendations for outpatient counseling and education.*

Questions Frequently Asked by Patients

1. CAN I GO BACK TO WORK?

Rates of return to work in heart failure patients depend on variables such as employment history, age, social stability, and severity of heart failure (NYHA Functional Class). An exercise stress test may be helpful in assessing a patient's capacity for activity.[10,11] Most patients are able to perform sedentary work which involves lifting a 10 pound maximum and occasionally lifting or carrying articles such as files or small tools. Some patients with mild heart failure may be able to perform jobs that require considerable walking or standing and involve lifting 20 pounds maximum. Patients with only mild aortic or mitral regurgitation, mild aortic or mitral stenosis, or mild hypertension may be able to lift up to 50 pounds occasionally.[12]

2. WHEN CAN I RETURN TO HOBBIES AND ACTIVITIES (LIKE SPORTS)?

An exercise test can assess exercise capacity and the likelihood of arrhythmias caused by physical activity.[12] A cardiac rehabilitation specialist or exercise physiologist can prescribe a personalized fitness regimen for patients. Patients with EF less than 35% may be at an increased risk for arrhythmias and pulmonary congestion. Exercise recommendations depend on factors such as severity of heart failure (NYHA class), previous procedures and interventions, valvular disease, medications, and left ventricular function.[13] You should advise patients to pace themselves and refrain from activities that cause an increase in symptoms with exercise.

3. WHAT ACTIVITIES SHOULD I AVOID?

Advise patients to avoid activities that cause them to become short of breath, light-headed, or fatigued. Advise them to stop any activity that increases their symptoms. Endurance sports should be avoided, as should activities that involve lifting heavy objects.[12]

4. WHAT FOODS SHOULD I LIMIT?

Patients should avoid foods high in sodium; salt should not be added to food. Patients should eat fresh foods (like fruits and vegetables) and avoid processed foods. They should limit alcohol consumption to no more than one drink per day. Patients with severe heart failure can consult a dietitian to obtain a specialized dietary plan.

5. How much salt can I have?

The answer to this question depends on the severity of the patient's heart failure. The Recommended Dietary Allowance (RDA) of sodium is 2400 milligrams, but patients with Class III–IV heart failure should limit their sodium intake to 2000 milligrams or less. Advise patients with severe or refractory heart failure to meet with a dietitian.

6. Is it safe for me to drive?

Patients who have a history of loss of consciousness due to an arrhythmia in general should not drive. Those who have symptomatic ventricular arrhythmia should be event free for six months before driving. Patients with nonsustained ventricular tachycardia who have had an AICD placed prophylactically for prevention of sudden death may drive.

7. What are the side effects of my medications?

Side effects depend on the type and dosage of the medications. See pages 178–179 for a table of commonly used medications and associated adverse reactions in patients with heart failure.

8. What happens if I miss a dose?

Encourage patients to take medications as prescribed. If they miss a dose, they should not compensate by doubling the next dose, but rather should take the next dose as indicated. If a gastrointestinal or febrile illness occurs, consult with a clinician before temporarily reducing doses of diuretics or vasodilators.

9. What tests are being done and why?

Patients with new onset or suspected heart failure should have a history and physical exam, lab (Chem 20, CBC, Urinalysis), ECG, and CXR. These will help determine if the presentation fits the diagnosis of heart failure. An echocardiogram will assess LV function and heart dimensions and is important in the diagnosis of etiology and severity of heart failure. Additional tests may be necessary subsequently.

10. How do I become involved in a support group?

If your hospital has a support group for heart failure patients, encourage the patient to contact the group coordinator. If your hospital does not provide this service, direct the patient to a nearby hospital that does have a support group for cardiac patients or suggest that he or she meet with a counselor who specializes in cardiac rehabilitation. Patients can also find heart failure forums and chat rooms on the Internet.

Potentially Difficult Questions that are Usually not asked, but Should Be:

1. How long am I going to live?

This is often a patient's most important question, and also the most difficult to answer. Estimates of patient prognosis can come from clinical trials.[14] Mortality rates per year for patient subgroups are as follows: NYHA Class II, 5-15%; NYHA Class III, 20-50%; and NYHA Class IV, 30-70%. In general, I emphasize that individuals can vary a great degree and, with adherence to medications and life-style recommendations, a patient's prognosis may be better than average.

2. How am I going to pay for medications/procedures?

Insurance companies pay for many medications and procedures for heart failure patients. Allow use of generic diuretics (for example, furosemide) when effective. Some pharmaceutical companies have patient medication assistance programs in cases of financial hardship (for instance, carvedilol, amiodarone).

3. Is the procedure going to hurt?

Reassure patients that the history and physical exam are painless. Virtually all patients will tolerate a small amount of blood being drawn for laboratory testing. Explain to patients that an echocardiogram is a non-invasive test that uses ultrasound to image the heart, similar to that performed routinely for women during pregnancy. Discuss with the patient the amount of pain they should expect with a cardiac catheterization and after major surgery such as coronary artery bypass graft (CABG) or valve replacement.

4. How long will I be in the hospital?

Hospital stays differ widely between patients and depend on the reason for hospitalization. Patients with heart failure should be discharged from the hospital when:

√ Symptoms of heart failure have been adequately controlled.
√ Reversible causes of morbidity have been treated or stabilized.
√ Patients and caregivers have been educated about medications, diet, activity and exercise recommendations, and symptoms of worsening heart failure.
√ Adequate outpatient support and follow-up care have been arranged.

Primary Prevention of Left Ventricular Dysfunction

Treatment of both hypertension and hypercholesterolemia can lead to the primary prevention of heart failure since hypertension and coronary artery diseases are leading causes of left ventricular dysfunction.[14] Findings from randomized controlled studies confirm that treatment of hypertension with stepped-care antihypertensive therapy,[15] or hypercholesterolemia with an HMG co-reductase inhibitor will reduce the new onset of heart failure.[16] Once heart failure is manifest, it is still important to keep these principles in mind for the secondary prevention of progression of heart failure.

Disease	Effect of Treatment on Incidence of Heart Failure
Hypertension[15]	↓ 49%
Hypercholesterolemia[16]	↓ 38%

In a recent retrospective analysis of 48,586 patients with known coronary artery disease, 44% had annual testing of low-density lipoprotein (LDL) cholesterol. Only 25% of these patients were at a target level of LDL less than 100 mg/dL, yet only 39% were taking lipid-lowering medication.[17]

ACE Inhibitors Can Prevent Progression to Heart Failure in Patients with Asymptomatic Left Ventricular Systolic Dysfunction

Even in the absence of symptoms, you should treat patients who have moderately or severely reduced left ventricular systolic function (ejection fraction ≤40%) with an angiotensin converting enzyme (ACE) inhibitor to reduce the subsequent likelihood of developing clinical heart failure.

Patients may have asymptomatic left ventricular dysfunction recognized prior to the development of clinical heart failure for a variety of reasons.

PATIENT CHARACTERISTICS THAT CAN LEAD TO THE IDENTIFICATION OF ASYMPTOMATIC LEFT VENTRICULAR DYSFUNCTION

- Post-MI
- Family history of cardiomyopathy
- Heart murmur
- Abnormal ECG
- Chest x-ray showing cardiomegaly

Summary of Pharmacologic Treatment of Left Ventricular Systolic Dysfunction

When initiating drug therapy of left ventricular systolic dysfunction, you should distinguish between treatment to correct patient symptoms and treatment to blunt disease progression.

Disease progression slows when treatment favorably affects structural changes of the heart. Biochemically mediated structural changes occur over a period of months to years and result from effects on myocytes or extracellular matrix.[18] Beneficial or adverse changes will result from the repertoire of proteins transcribed and translated from the cellular genome.[19] Neurohormonal activation or positive inotropic therapy that may help short-term symptoms may be deleterious if sustained in the long-term.

☑ *I initiate β-blocker therapy after patients are compensated on target doses of ACE inhibitors.*

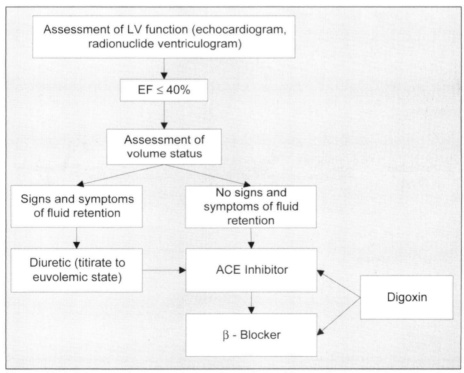

Figure 10-4. *Therapeutic approaches to the patient with systolic heart failure.* Reprinted from the American Journal of Cardiology with permission from Excerpta Medica Inc. M. Packer, Consensus recommendations for the management of chronic heart failure. On behalf of the membership of the advisory council to improve outcomes nationwide in heart failure, January 1999; 83:24A.[20]

Hemodynamic Effects of Vasoactive Medications in Heart Failure

Many drugs for the chronic therapy of heart failure affect either myocardial contractility, vascular tone, or both. In a given patient, the net effects of drug actions will determine the short-term result of therapy on hemodynamics and patient symptoms. As shown below, drugs that either *increase* contractility or *decrease* vascular tone will usually *increase* cardiac output. Drugs that *decrease* contractility or *increase* vascular tone will usually *decrease* cardiac output.

A low normal blood pressure (BP systolic 90-120 mm Hg) is appropriate for a patient with left ventricular dysfunction. When instituting disease progression treatment with either ACE inhibitors or β-blockade to avoid symptomatic hypotension, you may need to decrease a patient's dose of diuretics, thereby, increasing ventricular preload when using vasodilator drugs.

☑ *Hemodynamic effects of oral medications affect short-term symptoms.*

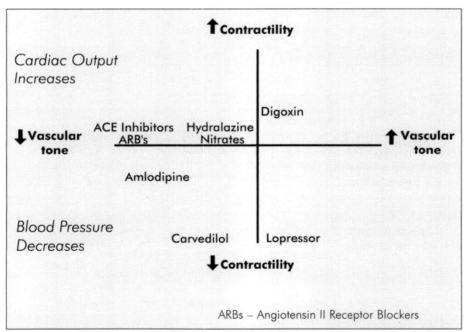

Figure 10-5. *Effects of commonly used oral medications on patient hemodynamics. For example, when initiated in heart failure, ACE inhibitors and angiotensin II receptor blockers usually increase cardiac output and decrease filling pressures.*

Outpatient Therapy for Volume Overload

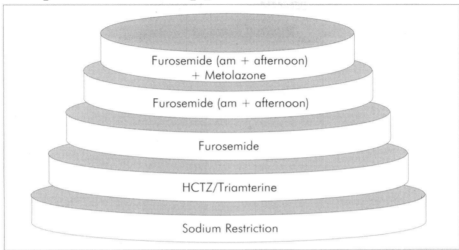

Figure 10-6. *Steps to outpatient therapy for volume overlaod.*

You should seek findings of volume overload in all patients with heart failure. You can manage some patients with mild volume overload adequately with sodium restriction and a thiazide diuretic. Most patients with congestion will require a loop diuretic such as furosemide.

Addition of metolazone 2.5-5 mg or hydrochlorthiazide 6.25-25 mg as a "booster" for loop diuretics can be added every one to three days. For recurrent hypokalemia, the aldosterone antagonist spironolactone (aldactone) 25-50 mg once or twice per day can be useful. The recently reported Randomized Aldactone Evaluation Study (RALES) found a 30% decrease in all cause mortality and a halving of hospitilizations in patients taking spironolactone — mean dose 26 mg per day — compared to placebo.[21] Blockade of non-renal effects of aldosterone on myocardial fibrosis or sympathetic nervous activity may be important since this dose has only a minimal diuretic effect.

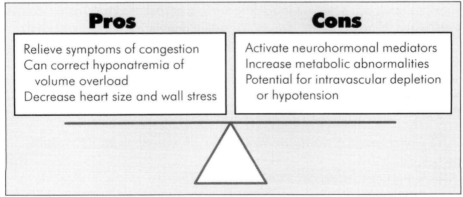

Figure 10-7. *Pros and cons of diuretics in heart failure.*

Loop Diuretics[22]

Generic Name	Brand Name	Equivalent Doses
furosemide	Lasix®	40 mg
bumetanide	Bumex®	1 mg
torsemide	Demadex®	20 mg
ethacrynic acid	Edecrin®	25 mg

☑ *An outpatient weight gain of three or more pounds should lead to an increase in diuretic dose.*

☑ *Most patients with heart failure will require a diuretic in addition to ACE inhibitor therapy.*

ACE Inhibitors

Patients with heart failure due to left ventricular systolic dysfunction should be given a trial of angiotensin converting enzyme (ACE) inhibitors unless specific contraindications exist: 1) history of intolerance or adverse reactions to these agents; 2) serum potassium greater than 5.5 mEq/L that cannot be reduced by diet or diuretic adjustment; or 3) symptomatic hypotension.[8] Patients with systolic blood pressure less than 90 mm Hg may still tolerate an ACE inhibitor, if managed by a clinician experienced in advanced heart failure. Caution and close monitoring are also required for patients who have a serum creatinine greater than 3.0 mg/dL or an estimated creatinine clearance of less than 30 mL/min; half the usual dose can be cautiously initiated in this setting.

ACE inhibitors can serve as initial therapy in the subset of heart failure patients who present with fatigue or mild dyspnea on exertion and who do not have any other signs or symptoms of volume overload. If symptoms of volume overload develop or persist, you should add a diuretic.

Although all ACE inhibitors lead to decreased production of angiotensin II, side effects may differ by specific agent. Any can lead to hypotension, cough, renal insufficiency, angioedema, and dysgeusia (change of taste). Those with sulfhydryl groups such as captopril may also cause neutropenia, rash, and proteinuria.[23]

☑ *Consider ACE inhibitor therapy in all patients with EF < 40%.*

☑ *Consider bilateral renal artery disease if ACE inhibitors precipitate marked renal insufficiency*

The Studies of Left Ventricular Dysfunction (SOLVD) Trial

MORTALITY IN ENALAPRIL VS. PLACEBO PATIENTS WITH NYHA CLASS II AND III HEART FAILURE

Use of the ACE inhibitor enalapril (10 mg po b.i.d.) in the Studies of Left Ventricular Dysfunction (SOLVD) trial in patients with heart failure symptoms and an EF less than or equal to 35%, showed an improvement in survival that began almost at the time of therapy. The difference between patients receiving enalapril versus placebo increased over time.[24]

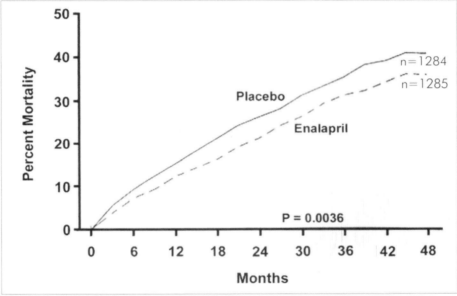

Figure 10-8. *SOLVD trial demonstrates an improvement in survival with enalapril therapy.* From The SOLVD Investigators. Effect of enalapril on survival in patients with reduced left ventricular ejection fractions and congestive heart failure. N.Engl.J.Med. 1991; 325:296. Reprinted with permission from The New England Journal of Medicine, copyright © 1991 Massachusetts Medical Society. All rights reserved.[24]

Reaching target doses of ACE inhibitor therapy can be important to achieve benefits found in multicenter trials. Decreasing the dose of diuretics may be necessary if hypotension occurs during titration of ACE inhibitor dose. Recently, a multicenter trial demonstrated a better efficacy of lisinopril 32.5-35 mg per day compared to 2.5-5.0 mg per day.[25]

☑ *If titration of ACE inhibitor therapy leads to hypotension prior to reaching target doses, consider reducing the dose of a patient's diuretic.*

Increasing Indications for ACE Inhibitors and Left Ventricular Dysfunction

The indications for use of ACE inhibitors for treatment of left ventricular dysfunction have increased over the last decade. Initially ACE inhibitors were evaluated for treatment of symptomatic left ventricular systolic dysfunction. Patients with Class II-IV heart failure treated with ACE inhibitors improved compared to placebo. Subsequently, ACE inhibitors were found to improve outcome for patients with left ventricular systolic dysfunction without overt symptoms of heart failure in three related categories of patients: first, asymptomatic patients with ejection fractions less than 35% due to either ischemic or non-ischemic cardiomyopathy[3]; second, patients 3-16 days following myocardial infarction with ejection fractions less than 40%[26]; third, patients presenting within the first 24- hours of myocardial infarction.[27,28]

In this last group, one strategy is to treat all patients who may tolerate ACE inhibitors without hypotension (BP_{sys} < 90) with ACE inhibitors initially. In patients after hospital discharge with preserved left ventricular ejection fraction (> 50%), my present practice is to discontinue ACE inhibitor therapy. Many of these patients will also receive chronic aspirin, cholesterol-lowering medication, and β- blockers. Others have suggested that all patients post-MI should be treated with ACE inhibitors indefinitely.

Why improvement is seen following initiation of ACE inhibitor therapy in patients with left ventricular dysfunction remains controversial.[29] The combination of the vasodilators isosorbide dinitrate and hydralazine also improves survival in heart failure, but not as much as ACE inhibitors.[30] Thus, both vasodilator and growth factor mechanisms may contribute to the favorable left ventricular remodelling and patient prognosis seen with ACE inhibitors.

Patient Subset	Drug	Study
Heart Failure		
Class II and III	enalapril	SOLVD[31]; V-HeFT II[30]
Class IV	enalapril	CONSENSUS[32]
Asymptomatic LV Dysfunction		
EF <35%	enalapril	SOLVD[3]
Post MI (EF <40%)	captopril	SAVE[26]
Acute MI	captopril, lisinopril	GISSI-3[27], ISIS-4[28]

SOLVD: Studies of Left Ventricular Dysfunction
V-HeFT: VA Heart Failure Trial
CONSENSUS: Cooperative North Scandinavian Enalapril Survival Study
SAVE: Survival and Ventricular Enlargement Trial

Following Acute Myocardial Infarction, the ACE Inhibitor Captopril Blunts Increases in LV End-diastolic Volume

Data from the Survival and Ventricular Enlargement Trial (SAVE) helped establish the relationship between cardiac structure and outcome. Both increased diastolic or systolic heart size by echocardiography at baseline assessment correlated with a worse survival in follow-up. Patients with the largest quartile of end-diastolic and end-systolic dimensions had an approximate 50% mortality over a three-year mean follow-up.[29]

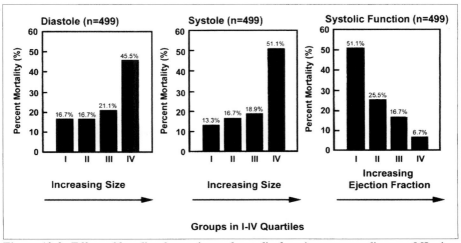

Figure 10-9. *Effect of baseline heart size and systolic function on mortality post-MI, ejection fraction < 40% (3-year mean follow-up).* Reproduced with permission. (M. St.John-Sutton, et al. Quantitative two-dimensional echocardiographic measurements are major predictors of adverse cardiovascular events after acute myocardial infarction. The protective effects of captopril. Circulation 1994; 89:71).[29]

Compared to placebo, patients who received the ACE inhibitor captopril had a blunting of increases in both left ventricular end-diastolic and end-systolic size. Preservation of heart size and structure at one year, was associated with a decrease in adverse cardiovascular events — cardiovascular death, heart failure requiring hospitalization, open label ACE inhibitor therapy, or recurrent myocardial infarction — from 31.8% with placebo to 20.7% with captopril during the mean follow-up of three years. These findings not only support the efficacy of ACE inhibitors for the treatment of left ventricular dysfunction, but also the broader hypothesis that measurable changes in left ventricular size and *structure* (disease progression) lead to changes in clinical outcome.

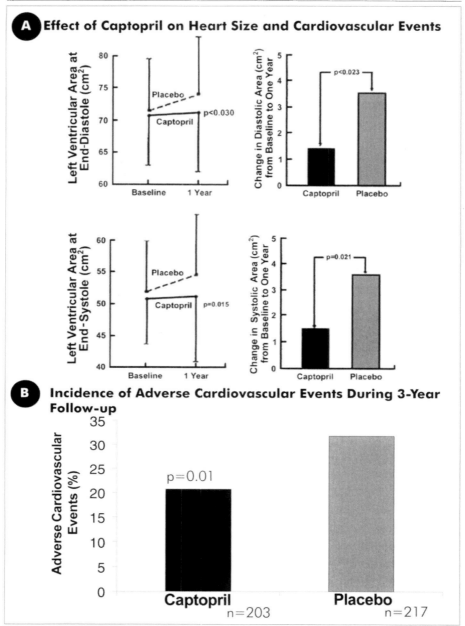

Figure 10-10. *The SAVE trial demonstrated that (A) ACE inhibitors blunt increases in heart size; prevention of ventricular enlargement at one year was associated with a reduction of cardiovascular events with captopril; and (B) Captopril reduced the incidence of adverse cardiovascular events during a 3-year follow-up.* Reproduced with permission. (M. St.John Sutton, et al. Quantitative two-dimensional echocardiographic measurements are major predictors of adverse cardiovascular events after acute myocardial infarction. The protective effects of captopril. Circulation 1994; 89:72).[29]

Angiotensin II Receptor Blockers (ARBs)

Angiotensin II receptor blockers (ARBs) may be an alternative when patients are intolerant of ACE inhibitor therapy. Use of either ACE inhibitors or ARBs will decrease the effects of angiotensin II (see pages 41–43); however, only ACE inhibitors block the degradation of and increase the levels of the vasodilator bradykinin. Although bradykinin may have beneficial effects including the release of nitric oxide and prostacyclin, it may also contribute to side effects such as angioedema and cough. Since ARBs do not affect bradykinin levels, these side effects are uncommon. With ACE inhibitor therapy, blockade of angiotensin II is still incomplete because alternate pathways also create an-

☑ *An increase in bradykinin is observed with ACE inhibitors, but not ARBs.*

giotensin II. Presently available ARBs block the angiotensin II, type-1 receptor (responsible for the direct cardiovascular effects of angiotensin II) and not the type-2 receptor (possibly a mediator for prevention of deleterious apoptosis). Thus, angiotensin II receptor blockers have effects related, but not equivalent to ACE inhibitors.[33]

In an initial comparison trial, Evaluation of Losartan in Treatment of the Elderly (ELITE), in patients with an ejection fraction less than 40 and age greater than 65 years, use of the ARB losartan was associated with a lower one-year mortality compared to the ACE inhibitor captopril.[34]

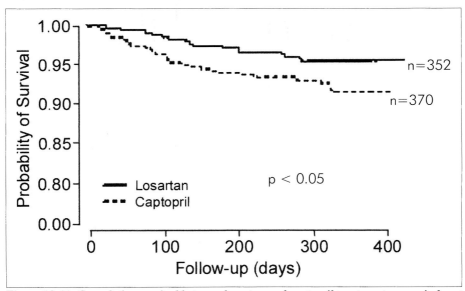

Figure 10-11. *Cumulative survival between losartan and captopril treatment groups in heart failure patients.* Reprinted with permission. Pitt B, et al. Randomised trial of losartan versus captopril in patients over 65 with heart failure (Evaluation of Losartan in the Elderly Study, ELITE). Vol. 349:750. © by the Lancet Ltd., 1997.[34]

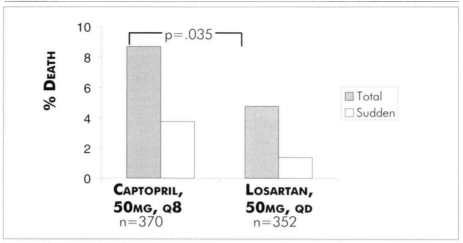

Figure 10-12. *Total and sudden death mortality in the ELITE trial.*[34]

A trend of a decrease in sudden death primarily accounted for the overall decrease in one-year mortality. The incidence of renal dysfunction, the primary endpoint of the trial, and hypotension related symptoms were similar with both classes of drugs.

In a preliminary report, the follow-up and larger ELITE II trial that randomized 3,152 patients to the same target doses of captopril versus losartan showed no statistically significant difference in the primary endpoint of all cause mortality (captopril 15.9% versus losartan 17.7%, NS) (see page 277). At present, patients with systolic dysfunction are candidates for angiotensin II receptor blockers if they:

1). Are intolerant of ACE inhibitors due to persistent cough or angioedema.
2). Have persistent hypertension despite ACE inhibitors and β-blockers.

Since production of angiotensin II persists despite use of ACE inhibitors, it has been proposed that *addition* of an angiotensin II receptor blocker to patients tolerating target doses of an ACE inhibitor may provide additional benefit. This breakthrough of angiotensin II formation is evident when assessing the hemodynamic effects of addition of the ARB, valsartan, to patients with heart failure on ACE inhibitors (Figure 10-13).[35] When the angiotensin II receptor blocker losartan was added to patients on ACE inhibitors, exercise capacity assessed by peak oxygen consumption and New York Heart Association functional class improved at six months compared to placebo.[36]

Several, large multicenter trials (ValHeFT: Valsartan Heart Failure Trial, and CHARM: Candesartan in Heart failure Assessment of Reduction in Morbidity and Mortality) are in progress to test the hypothesis that addition of the ARB to patients on ACE inhibitor therapy improves long-term prognosis.

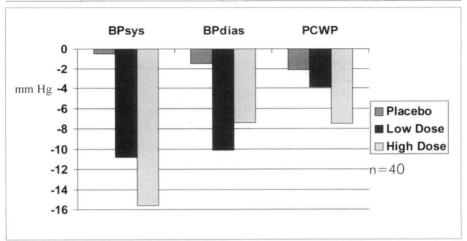

Figure 10-13. *Changes in hemodynamics with the addition of valsartan, an angiotension II blocker, in patients taking ACE inhibitors.*[35]

Additional Vasodilator Management

In patients with symptoms of heart failure despite target doses of ACE inhibitors, higher doses of ACE inhibitors (such as lisinopril, 40 mg po b.i.d.) have been reported to lead to additional symptomatic improvement.[37] This improvement was seen with a reduction in the severity of mitral regurgitation by Doppler echocardiography and reduction in left ventricular end-diastolic diameter. A decrease in symptoms, however, was unusual with marked left ventricular enlargement indicated by an end-diastolic diameter greater than 6.8 cm.

In patients with severe heart failure, inpatient treatment with the intravenous inotrope-vasodilator, milrinone, may facilitate up-titration of high-dose oral vasodilator therapy. In a study of 14 patients with severe heart failure and an ejection fraction of $18 \pm 6\%$, 10 who improved with milrinone were able to tolerate a 318% increase ACE inhibitor dose and survived for the subsequent 12 months. Four who did not respond to milrinone were unable to have doses similarly increased; two died within the 12 month follow-up period.[38]

Another alternative in patients with systolic dysfunction and contraindications or intolerance of ACE inhibitors is isosorbide dinitrate (20-40 mg) three times a day in combination with hydralazine (25-100 mg) three times a day (V-HeFT II).[39] When symptoms of low output predominate *despite* ACE inhibition, hydralazine can be added. Conversely, when symptoms of congestion predominate, nitrates may be a more effective drug to add.[40] Although not proven, isosorbide mononitrate (30-120 mg) once a day may be a more simple substitute for isosorbide dinitrate.

Sublingual Captopril vs. Sublingual Nitroglycerin

Similar to sublingual nitroglycerin, *sublingual* captopril (25 mg tablet) can acutely relieve shortness of breath due to pulmonary congestion.[41] Both agents increase cardiac output and decrease left ventricular preload and afterload. Compared to nitroglycerin, captopril has a slightly longer time to onset, but has a greater duration of action (over four hours). An additional dose of diuretics may be appropriate following either sublingual captopril or nitroglycerin to reduce the chance of recurrent symptoms. This therapy can avoid the need for emergency room treatment at night. Subsequently, however, heart failure patients should notify their clinician to reassess their status.

☑ *Both sublingual captopril and nitroglycerin may be useful to treat acute congestive symptoms.*

Hemodynamic Parameter	% Change After Treatment	(n=24) p-value vs. Baseline
CAPTOPRIL		
Cardiac Index	+ 49%	<.001
Pulmonary vascular resistance	− 42%	<.001
Systemic vascular resistance	− 33%	<.001
Mean blood pressure	− 16%	<.001
Mean pulmonary artery pressure	− 22%	<.001
NITROGLYCERIN		
Cardiac Index	+ 27%	<.001
Pulmonary vascular resistance	− 39%	<.001
Systemic vascular resistance	− 36%	<.001
Mean blood pressure	− 15%	<.001
Mean pulmonary artery pressure	− 19%	<.001

Figure 10-14. *Hemodynamic profiles of* sublingual *captopril and nitroglycerin.*[41]

The PRAISE Trial with Amlodipine

Use of calcium channel blockers in general have not led to an improved outcome in patients with heart failure. Acutely, calcium channel blockers have a mild direct negative inotropic effect that may be offset by left ventricular afterload reduction.[42] In clinical trials in patients with systolic dysfunction heart failure, the first generation calcium channel blockers, nifedipine, and diltiazem, were associated with an increase in adverse events.[43, 44] All calcium channel blockers are associated with some degree of fluid retention possibly related to intra-renal changes in blood flow and greater arterial compared to venous vasodilation.[45] Edema is common with nifedipine (short- or long-acting) but occurs with other agents as well. This effect may improve with better salt restriction and dose reduction.

The Prospective Randomized Amlodipine Survival Evaluation (PRAISE) trial showed no significant effect of amlodipine (10 mg per day) on survival in patients with ejection fractions less than 30%.[46] Surprising was the finding of a statistically significant survival benefit in the subgroup of patients with non-ischemic cardiomyopathy treated with amlodipine secondary to a decrease in both pump failure and sudden deaths.[47] The reason for this benefit is uncertain. Compared to placebo, amlodipine was associated with a slightly increased incidence of both pulmonary and peripheral edema. In a separate trial, no survival benefit was identified with the use of the related third generation dihydropyridine calcium channel blocker, felodipine (V-HeFT III).[48] Additional trials are in progress to specifically assess the use of amlodipine in patients with non-ischemic cardiomyopathy.

At this time, I reserve the use of amlodipine for patients who have systolic dysfunction and persistent hypertension despite target doses of ACE inhibitors, β-blocker therapy, and possibly hydralazine.

☑ *The target dose in the PRAISE trial was 10 mg of amlodipine.*

☑ *The goal of the PRAISE II trial will be to test the hypothesis that amlodipine improves outcome in patients with non-ischemic cardiomyopathy.*

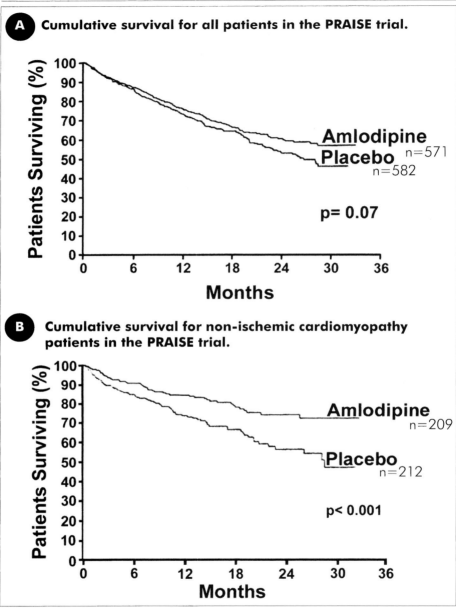

Figure 10-15. *The PRAISE Trial. (A) No significant effect of amlodipine on survival in patients with EF ≤ 30% was demonstrated. (B) Although not a primary endpoint, improved survival in the subgroup of patients with non-ischemic cardiomyopathy was observed with amlodipine.* From Packer M, et al. Effect of amlodipine on morbidity and mortality in severe chronic heart failure. Prospective Randomized Amlodipine Survival Evaluation Study Group. Vol. 335:1109.[46] Reprinted with permission from The New England Journal of Medicine, copyright © 1996 Massachusetts Medical Society. All rights reserved.

William Withering

(1741-1799)

William Withering was an English physician whose discovery of digitalis and his description of its use helped initiate clinical pharmacology.

Withering completed medical school at age 25 and entered general practice. He also developed an interest in botany, in part because his wife was an artist specializing in floral subjects. When he was 34 he was asked about a "secret by an old woman in Shropshire" who had a home remedy for a cure of "the dropsy" (fluid retention or edema). With his familiarity with botany, he was able to localize the active ingre-

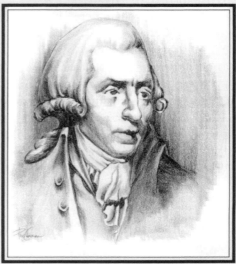

Figure 10-16. *William Withering.* Illustration by Peter Chapman.

dient as the foxglove leaf. Although Withering did not appreciate the significance as related to heart failure, he used this preparation as a diuretic.

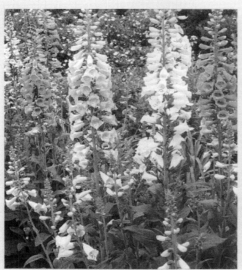

Figure 10-17. *The foxglove flower.*

Ten years later, Withering published his findings with digitalis, including effects on slowing the pulse and side effects when administered in toxic doses. He realized an association between an action on the "motion of the heart" and its benefits in some cases, but not all, as a diuretic. Further, he recognized that its effects would be more beneficial in patients who today we would recognize as having atrial fibrillation.

Withering's curiosity and subsequent careful clinical observations enabled other practitioners to apply his findings.

Digoxin

Controversy regarding the use of digitalis preparations, including digoxin, has persisted over the last 200 years.[49] It is a modest positive inotrope in patients with dilated left ventricles. It slows the rate of conduction of atrial fibrillation at the AV node of the heart. Finally, digoxin leads to a modest withdrawal of sympathetic tone in part by a direct effect on the baroreceptors within the carotid sinus. In patients with heart failure, afferent nerve traffic directed toward the brain's sympathetic control centers is often reduced. In animal models, this reduced nerve traffic increases with digoxin leading to a withdrawal of sympathetic nervous efferent traffic directed from the brain to the circulation. Electrical measurement of outflow of sympathetic nerve impulses decreases in patients with heart failure when given digoxin compounds, an effect not seen with dobutamine.[50]

The Digitalis Investigators Group (DIG) trial showed no difference in survival between patients with EF less than 45% randomized to receive digoxin (n=3397) versus placebo (n=3403).

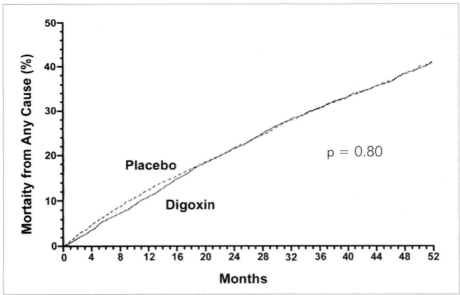

Figure 10-18. *DIG Trial, Placebo vs. Digoxin: Mortality from to any cause.* From The Digitalis Investigation Group. The effect of digoxin on mortality and morbidity in patients with heart failure. Vol. 336:527. Reprinted with permission from The New England Journal of Medicine, copyright © 1997 Massachusetts Medical Society. All rights reserved.[49]

The combined endpoints of death or hospitalization due to heart failure, however, were significantly reduced (Figure 10-19, p<0.001). There was a slight but statistically significant increase in the incidence of other cardiac deaths including sudden death not due to worsening heart failure in the digoxin group compared to placebo (15% vs. 13%, p=0.04, respectively).

Consider adding digoxin in patients with left ventricular systolic dysfunction who remain symptomatic despite ACE inhibitors and correction of volume overload. Since digoxin does not have an effect on overall mortality, patients with mild-to-moderate heart failure who are asymptomatic on optimal doses of ACE inhibitors and diuretics do not require digoxin. In a stable patient with heart failure, withdrawing digoxin may lead to worsening heart failure.[51]

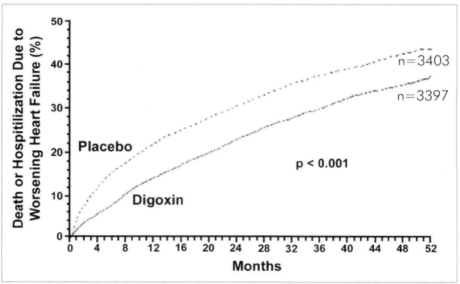

Figure 10-19. *DIG Trial, Placebo vs. Digoxin: Heart failure related death or hospitalization.* From The Digitalis Investigation Group. The effect of digoxin on mortality and morbidity in patients with heart failure. Vol. 336:527. Reprinted with permission from The New England Journal of Medicine, copyright © 1997 Massachusetts Medical Society. All rights reserved.[49]

☑ *Digoxin had no effect on overall patient survival.*

β-Blockers: The Metoprolol in Dilated Cardiomyopathy (MDC) Trial

Use of β-blockers for the treatment of either ischemic or non-ischemic cardiomyopathy has had a history of initial skepticism followed by gradual acceptance for treatment of disease progression in patients with mild or moderate heart failure.[52]

β-blockers can be classified as being first, second, or third generation based on specific pharmacologic properties. First generation β-blockers include propranolol which has non-specific blockade properties of both β_1 and β_2 catecholamine receptors. Second generation β-blockers include those that are specific for the β_1 receptor subtype such as metoprolol, bisoprolol, or atenolol. Third-generation β-blockers are those that have additional mechanisms of cardiovascular activity such as vasodilatation due to α-blockade. This last group would include carvedilol, bucindolol, and labetalol.

Trials assessed metoprolol in patients with non-ischemic dilated cardiomyopathy. Patients who tolerated metoprolol were found to have an increase in ejection fraction. This fit the paradigm of β-blockers preventing the adverse effects of catecholamines on myocyte function and structure due to chronic norepinephrine stimulation.

As shown in the Metoprolol and Dilated Cardiomyopathy trial, the combined endpoint of freedom from death or need for heart transplant was significantly reduced by metoprolol ($p < 0.01$). Nevertheless, mortality in this trial was not reduced by metoprolol.

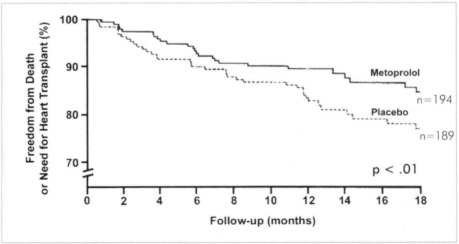

Figure 10-20. *Metoprolol in Dilated Cardiomyopathy (MDC) Trial.* Reprinted with permission. Waagstein F, et al. Beneficial effects of metoprolol in idiopathic dilated cardiomyopathy. Metoprolol in Dilated Cardiomyopathy (MDC) Trial Study Group. Vol. 342:1443. © by the Lancet Ltd., 1993.[52]

☑ *Metoprolol was the first β-blocker to show an improvement in ejection fraction in patients with non-ischemic cardiomyopathy.*

Other studies have documented an increase in β-receptor density both on myocytes and circulating lymphocytes following β-blockade with metoprolol. The initial hypothesis was that β-blockers were effective by blocking effects of catecholamines and returning cellular β-receptor phenotypes to a more normal level. This would reduce catecholamine stimulation of the heart but still allow an increase in responsiveness to transient elevation of catecholamines when needed. Recently, the Metoprolol Randomized Intervention Trial in Heart Failure (MERIT-HF)[53] found that sustained release metoprolol titrated to 200 mg per day compared to placebo decreased mortality 35% in patients with predominately NYHA Class II and III heart failure and an ejection fraction less than or equal to 40%.

Use of a similar second generation β-blocker, bisoprolol, was also associated with a 32% decrease in mortality compared to placebo in the Cardiac Insufficiency Bisoprolol Study (CIBIS II)[54] trial in patients with ischemic and non-ischemic cardiomyopathy.

Carvedilol

Carvedilol is a non-specific β_1 and β_2 receptor blocker with α-receptor blocker properties and antioxidant effects.[55] Whereas metoprolol leads to an increase in β-receptor density on myocytes, carvedilol maintains a low myocyte β-receptor density.[56]

In a series of four related trials in the United States in patients with ejection fractions less than 35%, carvedilol was associated with a 62% reduction in mortality (Figure 10-21) and an increase in ejection fraction seen over 6–12 months. Symptoms of heart failure were also significantly improved by both patient and physician assessment.[57] Whether carvedilol is more effective than metoprolol in improving heart failure disease progression is uncertain.[58,59] It is unknown whether more "complete" β-blockade without β-receptor upregulation is desirable. An ongoing direct comparison clinical trial will help determine the relative effects of carvedilol versus metoprolol on mortality in heart failure (Carvedilol or Metoprolol Evaluation Trial: COMET). Another third generation β-blocker, bucindolol, has non-specific β_1 and β_2 blockade and direct vasodilating effects. A large multicenter trial with this agent in heart failure (Bucindolol Evaluation of Survival Trial: BEST) showed no improvement compared to placebo.[60]

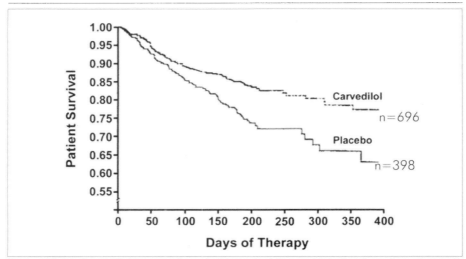

Figure 10-21. *Carvedilol improved survival in both patients with ischemic and non-ischemic cardiomyopathy.* Packer M, et al. The effect of carvedilol on morbidity and mortality in patients with chronic heart failure. U.S. Carvedilol Heart Failure Study Group. Vol. 334:1353. Reprinted with permission from The New England Journal of Medicine, copyright © 1996 Massachusetts Medical Society. All rights reserved.[57]

Effects of Carvedilol on Heart Size: Australia/New Zealand Trial

Whereas ACE inhibitors blunt increases in heart size following initial myocardial injury such as myocardial infarction, β-blockers may *reverse* myocardial enlargement when *added* to ACE inhibitor therapy.[61] In this study, carvedilol decreased end-systolic dimension and showed a trend to decrease end-diastolic dimension by echocardiography. Ejection fraction significantly increased (Figure 10-22). This effect on the structure of the heart in patients with heart failure supports the hypothesis that adverse consequences of ventricular enlargement are, in part, mediated by chronic excessive catecholamine stimulation.

Similarly, in 59 symptomatic patients with heart failure and an ejection fraction less than 35%, carvedilol led to other changes consistent with beneficial reverse remodeling after four months of therapy. Left ventricular mass, sphericity, and mitral regurgitation decreased by echocardiography and Doppler.[62]

TIPS FOR INITIATING β-BLOCKERS IN PATIENTS WITH HEART FAILURE

In general, compensated outpatients should be on target doses of ACE inhibitors prior to initiation of any β-blocker therapy. Low doses should initially be used with gradual titration to target doses to minimize symptoms of dizziness, fatigue, or worsening heart failure. Typically, if a patient is tolerating a β-blocker, the dose is doubled every 1–4 weeks until target doses are attained.

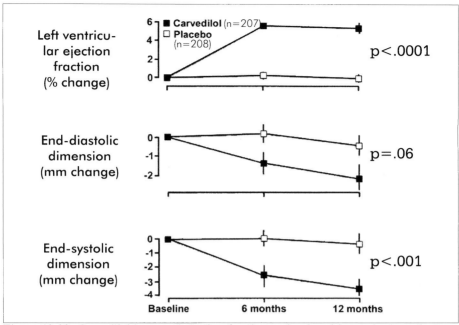

Figure 10-22. *Carvedilol improved ejection fraction and reduced heart size in patients on ACE inhibtor therapy.* Reprinted with permission. Australia/New Zealand Heart Failure Research Collaborative Group. Randomised, placebo-controlled trial of carvedilol in patients with congestive heart failure due to ischaemic heart disease. Vol. 349:377. © by the Lancet Ltd., 1997.[61]

Diuretics may require adjustment during the early phase of withdrawal of catecholamine stimulation. Dizziness, if due to hypotension, may improve with a reduction in diuretics. Shortness of breath, if due to pulmonary congestion, may require an increase in diuretics. If both occur, patients may not tolerate β-blockers. Data is limited on the use of β-blockers in patients with NYHA Class IV heart failure. If used after patient stabilization, these patients should receive close observation during initiation and titration of the drug.[63]

Chronic obstructive lung disease is common in elderly patients with heart failure, and it may be exacerbated by β-blockers. However, since the benefits of treatment are still potentially significant, I consider patients for β-blocker therapy who do not have severe lung disease by chest x-ray or active wheezing on physical exam. Although leg claudication due to peripheral artery disease may worsen with β-blockers, this is uncommon with carvedilol or metoprolol.

Whether β-blockers should be used in individuals with asymptomatic left ventricular dysfunction is unknown. First, some patients who deny symptoms have reduced their levels of activity to avoid symptoms and thus, are not actually asymptomatic. In the true absence of symptoms, I consider therapy for the younger or motivated individual to possibly achieve an increase in survival benefit.

Commonly Used Medications in Patients with Heart Failure

ACE inhibitors, the combination of isosorbide dinitrate and hydralazine, or β-blockers have been shown to reduce mortality in heart failure and thus blunt disease progression. Angiotensin II receptor blockers may have similar effects to ACE inhibitors.[8] Digoxin will not reduce mortality but improves symptoms of pump dysfunction and reduces the need for hospitalization for heart failure.

Drug	Initial Dose (mg)	Target Dose (mg)	Recommended Maximal Dose (mg)	Major Adverse Reactions
Thiazide Diuretics				
hydrochlorothiazide chlorthalidone	25 q.d. 25 q.d.	—	50 q.d. 50 q.d.	Postural hypotension, hypokalemia, hyperglycemia, increased uric acid, rash; rare severe reactions include pancreatitis, bone marrow suppression, and anaphylaxis
Loop Diuretics				
furosemide bumetanide ethacrynic acid torsemide	10-40 q.d. 0.5-1.0 q.d. 50 q.d. 10 q.d.	—	240 b.i.d. 10 q.d. 200 b.i.d. 100 b.i.d.	Same as thiazide diuretics
Thiazide-Related Diuretic				
metolazone	2.5 q.3.d.	—	10 q.d.	Same as thiazide diuretics
Potassium-Sparing Diuretics				
spironolactone triamterene amiloride	25 q.d. 50 q.d. 5 q.d.	—	100 b.i.d. 100 b.i.d. 40 q.d.	Hyperkalemia, especially if administered with ACE inhibitor; rash; gynecomastia (spironolactone only)

Legend:
q.d. —1x per day; b.i.d. — 2x per day; t.i.d. — 3x per day; q.i.d — 4x per day; q.3.d. — every third day

Drug	Initial Dose (mg)	Target Dose (mg)	Recommended Maximal Dose (mg)	Major Adverse Reactions
ACE Inhibitors				
lisinopril	5 q.d.	20 q.d.	40 b.i.d.	
enalapril	2.5 b.i.d.	10 b.i.d.	20 b.i.d.	Hypotension,
captopril	6.25-12.5 t.i.d.	50 t.i.d.	100 t.i.d.	hyperkalemia, renal
quinapril	5 q.d.	20 b.i.d.	20 b.i.d.	insufficiency,
ramipril	2.5 q.d.	10 q.d.	10 q.d.	cough, skin rash,
trandolapril	1 q.d.	4 q.d.	8 q.d.	angioedema,
fosinopril	10 q.d.	20 q.d.	40 q.d.	neutropenia
benazepril	5 q.d.	20 q.d.	40 q.d.	
digoxin	0.125- 0.25 q.d.	—	Serum level < 2.0 ng/ml	Cardiotoxicity, confusion, nausea, anorexia, visual disturbances
hydralazine	10-25 t.i.d.	75 t.i.d.	100 q.i.d.	Headache, nausea, dizziness, tachycardia, lupus-like syndrome
isosorbide dinitrate	10 t.i.d.	40 t.i.d.	80 t.i.d.	Headache, hypotension, flushing
isosorbide mononitrate	30 q.d.	60 q.d.	120 q.d.	Headache, hypotension, flushing
β-Blockers				
carvedilol	3.125 b.i.d.	25 b.i.d.	50 b.i.d.	Bradycardia,
metoprolol (extended release)	12.5 q.d.	200 q.d.	200 q.d.	dizziness, hypotension,
bisoprolol	1.25 q.d.	10 q.d.	10 q.d.	worsening heart failure
Angiotensin II Receptor Blockers				
losartan	25 mg q.d.	50 mg q.d.	100 mg q.d.	Dizziness, renal
valsartan	80 mg q.d.	160 mg q.d.	160mg q.d.	insufficiency,
irbesartan	150 mg q.d.	150 mg q.d.	300 mg q.d.	hypotension
candesartan	8 mg q.d.	16 mg q.d.	64 mg q.d.	

Legend:
q.d. —1x per day; b.i.d. — 2x per day; t.i.d. — 3x per day; q.i.d. — 4x per day

☑ *Titrating a patient to target doses of ACE inhibitors or β-blockers is desirable to reproduce the benefits demonstrated with these medications in multicenter trials.*

Treatment of Diastolic Dysfunction

Treatment of left ventricular diastolic dysfunction in the presence of pre-served systolic function remains a challenging problem.[64,65] Few trials of treatment of diastolic dysfunction are available; despite this, the following guidelines may help.

First, look for a treatable etiology of left ventricular diastolic dysfunction, especially coronary artery disease. Hypertrophic cardiomyopathy has unique clinical features that can affect therapy decisions and should lead to screening of genetically related individuals. At present, restrictive cardiomyopathy, either primary or due to amyloidosis, has no specific treatment, but uncovering the diagnosis can help to counsel a patient regarding prognosis or to anticipate other organ impairment. A patient with diastolic dysfunction due to hemochro-matosis or secondary iron overload can benefit from iron chelation therapy.

Second, titrate diuretics carefully. Elderly patients or others with intrinsic renal impairment can develop progressive pre-renal azotemia despite persistent vascular congestion. When this occurs, you can exclude renal artery stenosis by magnetic resonance angiography, radionuclide, or carbon dioxide angiography techniques.

☑ *Preload, afterload, and heart rate are targets for treatment of symptoms in diastolic dysfunction.*

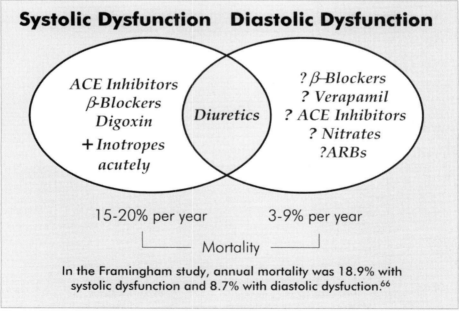

Systolic Dysfunction   Diastolic Dysfunction

ACE Inhibitors
β-Blockers
Digoxin
+ Inotropes
acutely

Diuretics

? β-Blockers
? Verapamil
? ACE Inhibitors
? Nitrates
?ARBs

15-20% per year   3-9% per year

└─── Mortality ───┘

In the Framingham study, annual mortality was 18.9% with systolic dysfunction and 8.7% with diastolic dysfuction.[66]

Figure 10-23. *Drug therapy of diastolic dysfunction. Circulatory congestion symptoms will improve with diuretics and possibly nitrates.*

Treatment of Diastolic Dysfunction Guided by Doppler Flow Pattern

TYPICAL CLINICAL FINDINGS

ABNORMAL RELAXATION	ABNORMAL DIASTOLIC COMPLIANCE
• Symptoms with activity • Inappropriate rapid heart rate • No detectable fluid overload • S_4 present on exam • Normal PR interval • Ventricular relaxation impaired by Doppler (Stage I)	• Symptoms at rest include orthopnea • Heart rate appropriate for degree of heart failure • Fluid overload • S_3 present on exam • Normal or prolonged PR interval • Diastolic compliance impaired by Doppler (Stage II, III, or IV)

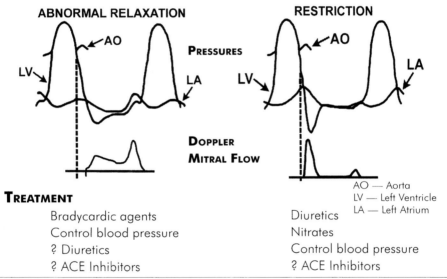

AO — Aorta
LV — Left Ventricle
LA — Left Atrium

TREATMENT

Bradycardic agents Control blood pressure ? Diuretics ? ACE Inhibitors	Diuretics Nitrates Control blood pressure ? ACE Inhibitors

Figure 10-24. *The use of Doppler flow pattern to guide treatment of diastolic dysfunction.* Above Doppler flows reprinted with permission from the American College of Cardiology (Journal of the American College of Cardiology, July 1997; 30:8-18).[67]

Third, control high blood pressure. Hypertensive heart disease is a common etiology for diastolic dysfunction usually with increased left ventricular wall thickness and calculated mass by echocardiography. Compared to the treatment of systolic dysfunction, the choice of antihypertensive agent may not be important. In hypertensive patients without heart failure, treatment with diuretics, β-blockers, calcium blockers or ACE inhibitors all led to similar decreases in calculated left ventricular mass by echocardiography.[68] Although it is logical to assume that a decrease in LV mass is a goal of antihypertensive treatment, it is unknown if left ventricular mass can serve as a surrogate measure for clinical improvement during therapy for diastolic dysfunction associated with left ventricular hypertrophy.

Fourth, treat atrial fibrillation. Left atrial enlargement commonly leads to atrial fibrillation and loss of atrial "kick." Atrial transport is important for maintaining adequate left ventricular preload in the patient with diastolic dysfunction. Sinus rhythm allows a physiologic increase in left ventricular end-diastolic pressure *without* an increase in pulmonary capillary wedge pressure.

Finally, in individuals with impaired early diastolic filling by Doppler, slowing heart rate can improve diastolic filling by increasing diastolic filling time. This is similar to treatment of impaired filling due to valvular mitral stenosis. By decreasing myocardial oxygen consumption, bradycardic medications also improve myocardial ischemia, a potential factor contributing to diastolic dysfunction. These mechanisms may contribute to improved function with β-blockers in patients with low ejection fraction, as well.

Obstructive vs. Nonobstructive Hypertrophic Cardiomyopathy

When patients with hypertrophic cardiomyopathy progress to findings of heart failure, therapy is appropriate to improve symptoms secondary to left ventricular outflow tract gradient and diastolic dysfunction.[69] β-blockers alone may be enough to improve symptoms, findings on physical exam, and/or hemodynamic testing. Diuretics may help symptoms of pulmonary congestion. However, they should be used carefully since they may increase outflow tract gradient by reducing left ventricular size. Digoxin is avoided.

Verapamil, a calcium channel blocker with negative inotropic effects, has also been used in hypertrophic cardiomyopathy. Because of its vasodilator effects, however, it can increase the outflow tract gradient in patients with obstructive cardiomyopathy. Nevertheless, verapamil can be considered second line treatment because of its bradycardic and negative inotropic effects similar to β-blockers. Although use of dihydropyridines such as nifedipine have been reported in hypertrophic cardiomyopathy, I avoid them because of their potent vasodilating effects and associated reflex tachycardia.

Amiodarone is the drug most commonly used for treatment of atrial or ventricular arrhythmias in hypertrophic cardiomyopathy. It also acts similarly to a β-blocker with slowing of sinus rate and AV node conduction. It is a moderate negative inotrope, potentially decreasing outflow tract obstruction.

Disopyramide may be considered a second line agent because of its antiarrhythmic and negative inotropic properties. This is potentially a useful drug when paroxysmal atrial fibrillation occurs and long-term side effects of amiodarone are not desired. Generally, disopyramide is given in patients already on β-blockers since alone it may increase the rate of atrial fibrillation.

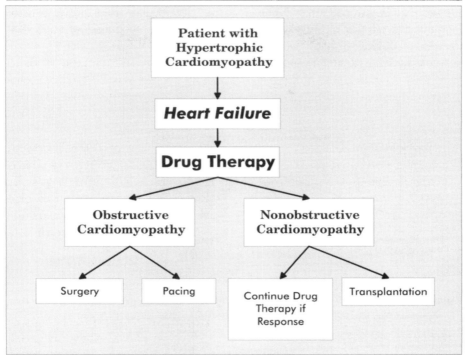

Figure 10-25. *Therapy of hypertrophic cardiomyopathy.*[69]

AV sequential pacing has been applied in patients with hypertrophic cardiomyopathy and left ventricular outflow tract obstruction. The mechanism of gradient reduction is not fully understood. Pacing the right ventricular apex may blunt high septal thickening into the left ventricle. In a controlled trial comparing pacing and no pacing, however, only a 25% decrease in outflow gradient with AV pacing was observed.[70] In general, preempting normal ventricular activation with pacing is desirable and is achieved by using a short AV pacing coupling interval.[71] In another randomized crossover study in patients with drug refractory symptoms, only a small subset of patients greater than or equal to 65 years of age responded clinically to AV pacing.[72]

Definitive treatment of obstructive hypertrophic cardiomyopathy in patients with refractory symptoms despite medical therapy is surgical myotomy-myectomy.[73] This therapy includes a septal wedge resection and incision to reduce septal contraction. Reported mortality at experienced centers with this procedure is between 1-2%.[69] It is unknown whether myotomy-myectomy improves the diastolic compliance abnormality of hypertrophic cardiomyopathy. Effects on sudden death rates are also not known. Severe mitral regurgitation and the outflow tract gradient associated with hypertrophic cardiomyopathy can improve with replacement of the mitral valve with a low profile mechanical valve (St. Jude® or Carbomedics®). Infusion of alcohol via an angioplasty catheter placed in a septal artery has been proposed as an alternative non-operative technique to achieve septal myocardial ablation.[74] In a recent series, mean left ventricular outflow gradient was reduced from 62 to 19 mm Hg with 21 of 25 patients showing clinical improvement.[75]

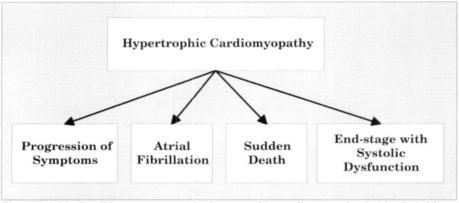

Figure 10-26. *Possible states caused by hypertrophic cardiomyopathy.* Spirito P, Seidman CE, McKenna WJ, Maron BJ. The management of hypertrophic cardiomyopathy. Vol. 336:779. Reprinted with permission from The New England Journal of Medicine, copyright © 1997 Massachusetts Medical Society. All rights reserved.[69]

In patients with symptomatic nonobstructive cardiomyopathy, treat diastolic dysfunction with medication until refractory symptoms result in the need for cardiac transplant if the patient is an appropriate candidate for this procedure. Aggressive prevention and treatment of atrial fibrillation is necessary in nonobstructive cardiomyopathy.

A small number of patients progress from hypertrophic cardiomyopathy with normal or hyperdynamic systolic function to dilated cardiomyopathy. The etiology of this transition is not known, but in general, is an advanced finding associated with a poor prognosis. Treatment with ACE inhibitors, diuretics, and digoxin remain appropriate at this stage until the patient is potentially a candidate for cardiac transplant.

In patients who have life threatening ventricular tachycardia or ventricular fibrillation, treatment with either an implantable defibrillator or amiodarone remain the two alternatives (similar to the treatment of ventricular arrhythmias in patients with dilated cardiomyopathy).[76]

Atrial Fibrillation and Heart Failure

Atrial fibrillation is common in heart failure. The onset of atrial fibrillation is associated with increasing size of the left atrium.[77] In patients with sustained atrial fibrillation, anticoagulation with warfarin to achieve a therapeutic international normalized ratio (INR) of 2-3 will reduce the incidence of subsequent embolic stroke.

Consider pharmacologic or electrical cardioversion when the duration of atrial fibrillation is known to be less than six months and left atrial size is less than 4.5 cm.[78] Patients should receive warfarin for three weeks prior to elective attempted cardioversion of chronic atrial fibrillation. If atrial fibrillation is of less than 48-hours duration, anticoagulation is not mandatory prior to cardioversion. Many class I antiarrhythmic agents have led to increased mortality in patients with left ventricular dysfunction and thus, are avoided.[79] Amiodarone, a class III agent with a biologic half-life of weeks, however, may be a useful adjunct to achieve or maintain sinus rhythm. With this, sinus rhythm after cardioversion may be maintained with a left atrial size up to 6 cm.[80] In patients with permanent atrial fibrillation, digoxin, β-blockers, and amiodarone can control ventricular response rate. I avoid the calcium channel blockers, diltiazem and verapamil, to slow ventricular response with left ventricular systolic dysfunction since fluid retention may increase without effect on heart rate in this setting. Chemical cardioversion with rapid acting IV agents (such as ibutalide) is less effective in patients with heart failure and may precipitate ventricular arrhythmia.

Refractory patients with atrial fibrillation and a rapid ventricular response despite medical therapy can undergo catheter based radiofrequency ablation of the AV node with placement of a rate responsive permanent ventricular pacemaker. Doing so can improve symptoms of palpitations, dyspnea, exercise intolerance, fatigue, and chest pain.[81]

☑ *If atrial fibrillation is of more than 48-hours duration, consider anticoagulation prior to electrical cardioversion.*

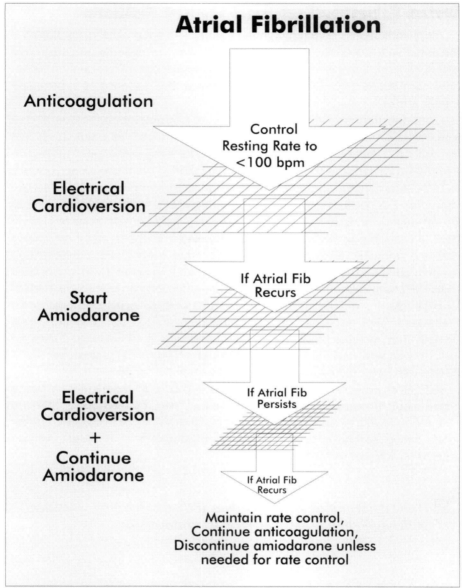

Figure 10-27. *Atrial fibrillation and heart failure: progression of treatment.*

☑ *Consider urgent cardioversion if a patient is hemodynamically unstable because of rapid atrial fibrillation, even if duration is unknown.*

Amiodarone

Clinicians experienced with using amiodarone should initiate therapy because of the long half-life and potential for toxicity of the drug.[82]

Amiodarone	
Effect on ECG	• Action potential duration increased • Sinus rate decreased • PR interval increased • Rate of conduction of atrial fibrillation decreased • Ventricular ectopy decreased
T$_{1/2}$	• 40-55 days

Drug Interactions	• Increases effect of warfarin and levels of digoxin, theophylline
	  Use cautiously with other bradycardiac agents
	  (β–blocker, Ca^{++} channel blocker)

☑ *If a heart failure patient is on diltiazem or verapamil for rate control of atrial fibrillation, consider changing to amiodarone.*

Amiodarone, in part, acts as a sympatholytic agent at the heart by reducing the release of norepinephrine from cardiac sympathetic nerves.[83] β-blockers and amiodarone can be used together; however, this may be limited by bradycardia.[84]

Type of Arrhythmia	Common Doses
Atrial Arrhythmias	*Oral:* • 400 mg b.i.d. x 1 week • 200 mg b.i.d. x 3+ weeks • 200 mg q.d. (may vary)
Ventricular Arrhythmias	*Oral:* • 600 mg b.i.d. x 1 week • 400 mg b.i.d. x 3 weeks • 200 mg b.i.d.
Acute Life Threatening Arrhythmias	*IV:* • 150 mg over 10 min, may repeat • 1 mg/min x 6 hours • 0.5 mg/min subsequently

☑ *Some patients with atrial fibrillation may require higher chronic doses of amiodarone to maintain sinus rhythm.*

POSSIBLE SIDE EFFECTS OF AMIODARONE*

- Pulmonary inflammation
- GI
- Abnormal LFT's
- Nausea
- Neuropathy
- Rash or photosensitivity
- Hyper- or hypothyroidism
- Asymptomatic corneal deposits
- Proarrhythmia
  * *Dose related side effects are uncommon at doses < 300 mg/day*

Before starting amiodarone, a baseline thyroid panel and liver function panel should be obtained. Serum levels of amiodarone can be obtained, but are not useful for titration of dose. If low, they can indicate low absorption or noncompliance.

Assessment and Treatment of Ventricular Arrhythmias Associated with Left Ventricular Dysfunction

AMIODARONE VS. AICD

In patients who have manifest sustained ventricular tachycardia or ventricular fibrillation, when treatable secondary causes have been excluded, patients will survive longer with placement of an automatic implantable cardioverter defibrillator.[85] Whether patients with high-grade ventricular arrhythmias or with a low ejection fraction alone benefit from a transvenous automatic implantable cardioverter defibrillator (AICD) is uncertain. In patients with ischemic cardiomyopathy and spontaneous nonsustained ventricular tachycardia, a subset of these patients may benefit from prophylactic AICD placement as suggested by the Multicenter Automatic Defibrillator Implantation Trial (MADIT).

The MADIT Trial was the first study to show that sudden death could be prevented in a high risk subgroup of patients with ischemic cardiomyopathy (ejection fraction ≤35%) prior to an episode of life threatening arrhythmia. All patients had a history of a Q-wave myocardial infarction occurring greater than three weeks before entry associated with a documented episode of asymptomatic nonsustained ventricular tachycardia between 3-30 beats total at a rate of greater than 120 beats per minute. Patients were eligible for randomization only if they failed suppression with procainamide of an arrhythmia induced by an electrophysiologic study.

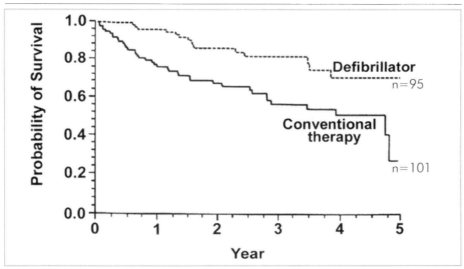

Figure 10-28. *The MADIT trial showed a higher probability of survival with an automatic implantable cardiac defibrillator (AICD) over conventional therapy in patients with ischemic cardiomyopathy and spontaneous nonsustained ventricular tachycardia.*[86] From Moss AJ, et al. Improved survival with an implanted defibrillator in patients with coronary disease at high risk for ventricular arrhythmia. Multicenter Automatic Defibrillator Implantation Trial Investigators. Vol. 335:1938. Reprinted with permission from The New England Journal of Medicine, copyright © 1996 Massachusetts Medical Society. All rights reserved.

Although the results of this trial have been disputed because of differences in medications between the two groups, the difference in outcome and prevention of sudden death is striking. This was despite half the patients in the defibrillator group receiving their defibrillator through a higher risk transthoracic approach compared to the current standard transvenous approach. Sudden death prevention by use of AICD devices is undergoing additional clinical trials.

Anticoagulation

Warfarin anticoagulation is indicated in patients with chronic atrial fibrillation or history of pulmonary or systemic thromboembolism. My practice is to also anticoagulate any patient with a history of left ventricular thrombus identified by echo or left ventriculography.

Recently a multivariate analysis of the SOLVD Trial (see page 46) found a statistically significant 24% decrease in risk of death or hospital admission in heart failure patients on warfarin, independent of the presence of atrial fibrillation, age, ejection fraction, or other variables.[87] In the absence of definitive trial data, I recommend using warfarin in younger patients with more advanced findings of heart failure. In patients with ischemic left ventricular dysfunction, I discontinue aspirin when I initiate warfarin.

Heart Failure Clinic

Symptoms of heart failure are potentially recurrent and disabling. Up to 40% of heart failure patients 70 years or older admitted to the hospital will require repeat hospital admission within 90 days.[88] New paradigms using "low-tech" approaches, including a heart failure clinic, can complement "high-tech" approaches to reduce the disability associated with chronic heart failure. Programs that encourage patient education and appropriate use of medical resources can improve patient symptoms and possibly long-term outcome.

An advanced nurse clinician as a team member focused on clinical issues affecting the heart failure patient can provide care beyond that usually achieved by a physician alone. Data base assessment of group patient outcomes can identify trends in patient care that require additional attention.

Telemanagement can prevent the need for patient hospitalization. Telephone monitoring especially to identify an increase in weight, treatable with an increase in diuretics, is an important component of heart failure clinic therapy resulting in a decreased need to hospitalize patients.[89]

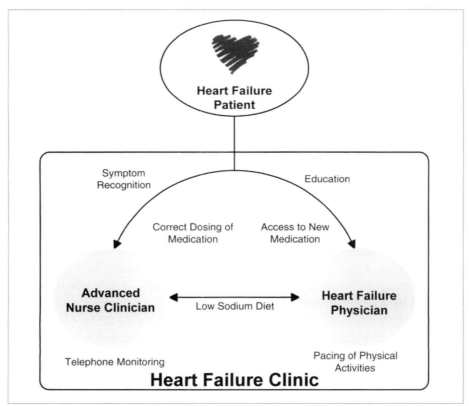

Figure 10-29. *The heart failure clinic can provide comprehensive care by combining high-tech and low-tech approaches to treatment.*

At the University of California Los Angeles Medical Center heart failure clinic, 214 patients with Class III to IV heart failure awaiting cardiac transplant had a marked reduction in hospitalization after enrollment.[90] This represented an 85% reduction in hospitalization associated with improvement in functional status as assessed by both symptom functional class and peak oxygen consumption. Estimated savings in hospital readmission costs was $9,800 per patient.

This remarkable improvement in clinical outcome over a six month period was achieved by adjusting patient therapies: ACE inhibitor doses on average were doubled; oral nitrates were increased; diuretic doses were increased; digitalis use was increased; antiarrhythmic agents were reduced (except for amiodarone which was increased); and calcium channel blockers were reduced. β-blocker therapy was not available for the treatment of heart failure during this series; additional benefits would be expected with this therapy.

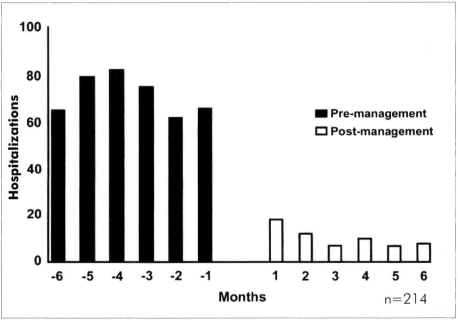

Figure 10-30. *Hospitalizations per month, before and during patient participation in the UCLA heart failure clinic.* Reprinted with permission from the American College of Cardiology (Journal of the American College of Cardiology, September 1997; 30:729).[90]

Referral or Consideration for Cardiac Transplantation

If patients remain symptomatic despite maximum medical therapy, consider consulting with a cardiologist who has expertise in the management of heart failure, if this has not been done previously.

Consider referral for cardiac transplantation evaluation in patients with significant exercise limitation or repeated hospitalizations because of heart failure — despite aggressive medical therapy in whom other interventions are unlikely to convey benefit. Generally, patients are 65 years or younger in age.

Measurement of patient oxygen consumption during cardiopulmonary exercise testing can provide useful prognostic information to aid with the timing of listing for cardiac transplantation. A peak O_2 consumption of less than 14 ml O_2/kg/min can indicate a poor one-year prognosis with continued medical therapy (Figure 10-32).[91] Especially in patients younger than 40 years old, percent predicted peak O_2 consumption (PPVO$_2$ corrected for age, body size, and sex) less than 50% can identify a worse prognosis than a single value threshold of 14 ml O_2/kg/min (Figure 10-33). Conversely, a peak O_2 consumption greater than 50% than predicted, led to a one- and two-year survival of 98% and 90%.[92] Both peak O_2 consumption and PPVO$_2$ are used in practice.

In heart failure patients with a reduced exercise capacity, use of a modified Naughton treadmill protocol allows a longer period of exercise to estimate peak oxygen consumption compared to protocols that increase workload at a more rapid rate such as the Bruce protocol. In the modified Naughton protocol each stage increases estimated O_2 consumption by 1 MET (3.5 ml O_2/kg/min) (Figure 10-31).

The occurrence of cardiac cachexia defined as a non-intentional weight loss of at least 7.5% over six months is an ominous finding associated with a 39% one-year mortality[93] and an independent risk factor for death. This finding should also lead to consideration for cardiac transplantation.

MODIFIED NAUGHTON		
Stage	MPH	% Grade
I	1.0	0
II	1.5	0
III	2.0	3.5
IV	2.0	7.0
V	2.0	10.5
VI	3.0	7.5
VII	3.0	10.0
VIII	3.0	12.5
IX	3.4	12.0
X	3.4	14.0

1 Stage = 2 minutes

Figure 10-31. *Example of modified Naughton protocol useful for exercise testing in patients with heart failure.*[94]

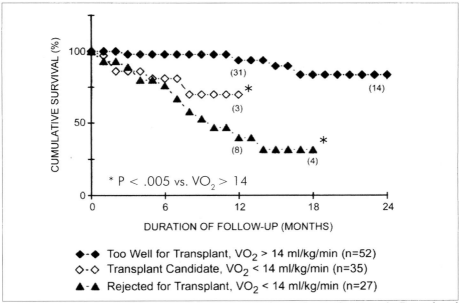

Figure 10-32. *Peak VO₂ with cardiopulmonary exercise testing and prognosis.* Reproduced with permission (D.M. Mancini, et al. Value of peak exercise oxygen consumption for optimal timing of cardiac transplantation in ambulatory patients with heart failure. Circulation 1991; 83:781).[91]

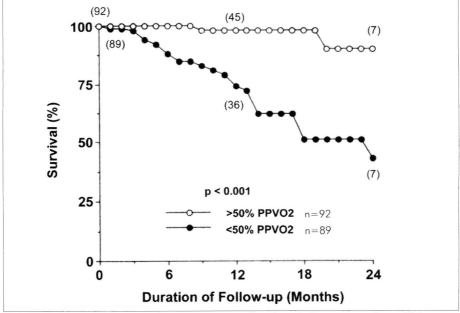

Figure 10-33. *In younger patients, percent predicted peak O₂ consumption will be more likely to predict a poor prognosis.* Reprinted with permission from the American College of Cardiology (Journal of the American College of Cardiology, February 1996; 27:348).[92]

Principal Developments in Cardiac Transplantation

Experimentation and development of cardiac transplant as a therapeutic procedure for end-stage heart failure has occurred over the last century. Dr. Alex Carroll published initial animal techniques for anastomosis of a heart from one dog to another in 1906. No human attempts were possible, however, until basic techniques of cardiac surgery evolved including the use of the heart/lung bypass machine. In 1960, Dr. Norman Shumway achieved the first long-term survival in a dog animal model with the dog surviving for eighteen days. His grafting technique of surgery including an atrial to atrial anastomosis is still used today. Finally, in 1967, Dr. Christian Bernard in Capetown,

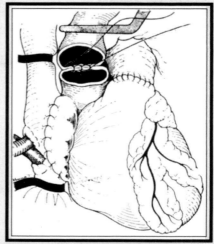

Figure 10-34. *Heart transplantation.* Illustration reprinted with permission from W.B. Saunders Company: J. Wallwork, Heart and Heart-Lung Transplantation, Copyright 1989.

South Africa followed shortly thereafter by Dr. Norman Shumway in the United States, achieved the first results in humans using human donor hearts. "Orthotopic" cardiac transplant is performed with the heart of the donor placed in the correct or replacement position of a recipient's heart (ortho — right, true).

Initially, outcome following cardiac transplant was poor with less than 40% one-year survival. Development of techniques of transvenous endomyocardial biopsy allowed diagnosis of rejection prior to graft failure. The availability of donor hearts increased by application of distant donor heart procurement techniques with safe transport ischemic times of at least four hours.

The current era of cardiac transplantation in 1980 began with the clinical use of the immunosuppressant cyclosporine A. Cyclosporine, which specifically suppresses T-helper cell function by blocking the effects of the cytokine interleukin II, increased survivial associated with a decrease in both rejection and infection.

Most patients following heart transplant are returned to a New York Heart Association Class I functional status, although peak exercise capacity and oxygen consumption are less than matched controls.

Cardiac transplant is a mature intervention limited by the availability of donor organs. At present, approximately 2000 heart transplants per year occur in the United States. Recent alternatives for immunosuppression include the use of mycophenolate mofetil[95] and tacrolimus.[96]

YEAR	EVENT
1906	Carrel: Proposed heart transplant techniques
1960	Shumway: Dog model of orthotopic transplant
1967	Bernard: Successful heart transplant in man
1968	Shumway: Successful heart transplant in United States
1972	Endomyocardial biopsy
1977	Distant donor heart procurement
1980	Cyclosporine-A

Cause of Death Following Cardiac Transplant (1985-1995)

Following heart transplant, the etiology of patient death varies with the time following heart transplant.[97] In the first month, graft failure due to either non-immune mechanisms or hyperacute rejection without inflammatory cell infiltrates of rejection predominate. Some of these patients may be bridged to repeat heart transplant with use of a mechanical support device.

Between one month and twelve months following heart transplant, infection and cellular rejection are the major reasons for patient death. During this time interval, an accelerated coronary artery atherosclerosis syndrome, in part a manifestation of chronic graft rejection, also becomes evident.

Beyond one year, graft atherosclerosis is the leading cause of death following heart transplant. Finally after five years, malignancy becomes a greater concern. Malignancies that are characteristic for the patient on chronic immunosuppression include lymphoma, lung cancer, and rapidly progressive skin cancers.

☑ *Patient survival following cardiac transplantation*[97]

1 year = 85%
5 year = 67%
10 year = 40%

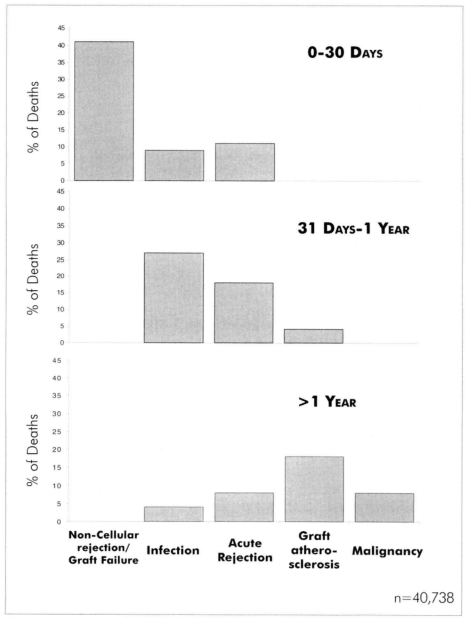

Figure 10-34. *Causes of death following cardiac transplantation. Data from 1985-1995.*[97]

Chapter 10 Case Scenarios

SCENARIO #1

MEDICAL HISTORY
77-year-old female with a history of ischemic cardiomyopathy (EF = 35%) with afternoon fatigue. History of severe asthma.

MEDICATIONS
lisinopril, aspirin

PHYSICAL EXAM
110/70 90 reg
Neck veins flat
Lungs: clear
2/6 Systolic Ejection Murmur (SEM) S_3
No edema

Question 1

What would you recommend for this patient?

a) losartan

b) isosorbide dinitrate & hydralazine

c) digoxin

d) amlodipine

e) carvedilol

SCENARIO #2

MEDICAL HISTORY
67-year-old male with a history of ischemic cardiomyopathy (EF = 25%) with stable fatigue on climbing one flight of stairs. No angina, orthopnea.

MEDICATIONS
lisinopril, digoxin, furosemide, K⁺, simvastatin, aspirin

PHYSICAL EXAM
110/70 90 reg
Neck veins flat
Lungs: clear
2/6 SEM S_3
Trace edema

Question 2

What would you recommend for this patient?

a) losartan

b) isosorbide dinitrate & hydralazine

c) digoxin

d) amlodipine

e) carvedilol

SCENARIO #3

MEDICAL HISTORY
79-year-old male with a history of ischemic cardiomyopathy (EF = 23%) with increased creatinine of 3.0. Intermittent shortness of breath at rest.

MEDICATIONS
lisinopril, digoxin, furosemide, K$^+$, aspirin

PHYSICAL EXAM
110/70 90 reg
Neck veins flat
Lungs: clear
2/6 SEM S$_3$
Trace edema

Question 3

What would you recommend?

a) losartan

b) isosorbide dinitrate & hydralazine

c) amiodarone

d) amlodipine

e) carvedilol

SCENARIO #4

MEDICAL HISTORY
59-year-old female with a history of non-ischemic cardiomyopathy (EF = 28%) with mild dyspnea on climbing two flights of stairs.

MEDICATIONS
lisinopril, digoxin, furosemide, K$^+$, carvedilol

PHYSICAL EXAM
165/90 60 reg
Neck veins flat
Lungs: clear
2/6 SEM S$_3$
No edema

Question 4

What would you recommend?

a) losartan

b) isosorbide dinitrate & hydralazine

c) amiodarone

d) amlodipine

e) warfarin

SCENARIO #5

MEDICAL HISTORY
63-year-old female with a history of non-ischemic cardiomyopathy
(EF = 31%) with persistent non-productive cough despite increased
doses of furosemide.

MEDICATIONS
lisinopril, digoxin, carvedilol,
furosemide, K^+

PHYSICAL EXAM
110/70 90 reg
Neck veins flat; no abdominojugular reflux
Lungs: clear
2/6 SEM S_3
No edema
CXR: Cardiomegaly, no pulmonary congestion

Question 5

What would you recommend for this patient?

a) losartan

b) isosorbide dinitrate & hydralazine

c) amiodarone

d) amlodipine

e) warfarin

See Appendix for solutions.

Inpatient Therapy

Chapter 11

Patients with worsening or advanced heart failure may require inpatient therapy. This chapter examines the therapeutic strategies for decompensated individuals. Attention is given to pulmonary congestion, pharmacologic management, mechanical assistance, and possible future directions of heart failure management.

Worsening Heart Failure vs. Other Cardiac Events Leading to Hospital Admission

When a patient with heart failure develops new or worsening symptoms, it is useful to begin with an assessment of the primary reason for decompensation:

PRIMARY REASONS FOR DECOMPENSATION

1). Worsening heart failure

2). Other cardiac events — arrhythmias or myocardial ischemia

3). Non-cardiac disease — pneumonia, gastrointestinal bleeding, etc.

Since the primary occurrence of any one of these conditions can lead to secondary exacerbation of other conditions, it is common for patients to present with multiple manifestations of disease. Discovering the primary reason for patient symptoms, such as acute myocardial infarction, can focus initial priorities for therapy, although treatment is usually necessary for both primary and secondary factors.

☑ *Determination of the primary factors for decompensation determines initial therapy.*

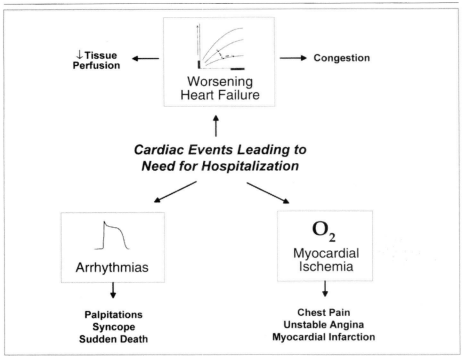

Figure 11-1. *Cardiac causes of hospitalization include worsening heart failure, arrhythmias, and myocardial ischemia.*

Precipitating Factors of Worsening Heart Failure

While treating acute symptoms, identification of precipitating factors is important in patients with known LV dysfunction. If the patient has severe findings of heart failure then intravenous therapy with nitrates (nitroglycerin, nitroprusside), phosphodiesterase inhibitors (milrinone), dobutamine, or dopamine may be appropriate.

PRECIPITATING FACTORS FOR HEART FAILURE

- Infection
- Arrhythmia (for example, atrial fibrillation)
- Myocardial ischemia
- Noncompliance of patient with medical regimen
- Toxic drug use

☑ *Identifying precipitating factors is important in decompensated chronic heart failure.*

OBJECTIVES AND PRIORITIES - SYMPTOM RELIEF

OBJECTIVES
1. Maintain cardiac function
2. Correct metabolic abnormalities
3. Identify and treat precipitating factors

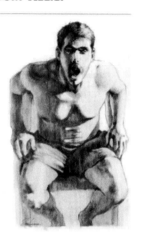

PRIORITIES
1. Hemodynamics
2. Arrhythmias
3. Neurohormonal Status

Figure 11-2. *Decompensated heart failure objectives and priorities.* Illustration by Peter Chapman.

DRUGS THAT CAN EXACERBATE HEART FAILURE[1]

- **Class I antiarrhythmics**
  (e.g., procainamide, quinidine, disopyramide, flecainide)

- **Calcium channel blockers**
  (if used for atrial fibrillation, consider amiodarone)

- **Non-steroidal anti-inflammatory drugs**
  (e.g., indomethacin, naproxen)

- **Alcohol or illicit drugs**
  (e.g., cocaine, amphetamines, etc.)

☑ *Discontinue medications that can exacerbate heart failure.*

When patients receiving outpatient β-blockers present with decompensated heart failure, consider decreasing the dose if only mild, low output, or congestion findings are present. For profound decompensation, discontinue β-blockers and resume them at low dose with cautious up-titration when patients are compensated.

Hospital Admission Guidelines

In the patient who requires hospital admission, diagnosis and therapy must often begin together. During the admission, initial intravenous therapy is replaced by oral therapy after the treatment of precipitating factors. Discharge care should attempt to prevent recurrence via patient and family education, home health assessments, and/or additional oral medication.

No simple set of criteria can address all potential patient criteria for admission to the hospital. Some of the below manifestations may be successfully treated with outpatient therapy including administration of IV diuretics, or brief vasoactive drug infusions. These guidelines for hospital admission were developed by the Agency of Health Care Policy and Research.[2]

PRESENCE OR SUSPICION OF HEART FAILURE AND ANY OF THE FOLLOWING FINDINGS CAN INDICATE A NEED FOR HOSPITALIZATION

- Clinical or ECG evidence of acute myocardial ischemia
- Pulmonary edema or severe respiratory distress
- Oxygen saturation below 90% (not due to pulmonary disease)
- Severe complicating medical illness (e.g., pneumonia)
- Anasarca
- Symptomatic hypotension or syncope
- Heart failure refractory to outpatient therapy
- Inadequate social support for safe outpatient management

Hospital Discharge Guidelines

Similarly, discharge guidelines depend on the duration of the patient's symptoms and likelihood for recovery.[2] In patients with new onset heart failure, every effort should be made to identify either surgical or medical therapy that could lead to cure; for example, valve replacement. In the large group of patients without this option or with known chronic heart failure, return to a stable, compensated state is the goal.

For patients with end-stage heart failure, who are not candidates for cardiac transplant, quality-of-life issues predominate. After discussions with the patient and his/her family, the patient may want to consider a "do not attempt" cardiopulmonary resuscitation status or hospice care.

> **PATIENTS WITH HEART FAILURE SHOULD BE DISCHARGED FROM THE HOSPITAL WHEN:**
>
> - Symptoms of heart failure have been adequately controlled.
> - Reversible causes of morbidity have been treated or stabilized.
> - Patients and caregivers have been educated about medications, diet, activity and exercise recommendations, and symptoms of worsening heart failure.
> - Adequate outpatient support and follow-up care have been arranged.

Initial Testing

When a patient is hospitalized, it is important to identify acute myocardial infarction usually by patient history and ECG — since this normally indicates a need for immediate coronary angioplasty or intravenous thrombolysis. In addition to basic data, cardiac enzymes and arterial blood gases may be appropriate tests. You should consider obtaining a echocardiography-Doppler study if one has not been performed within the previous year. Further diagnostic testing usually will await initial treatment, hemodynamic stability, and general improvement.

☑ *Exclude acute MI in patients with new onset decompensated heart failure.*

Initial Treatment of Acute Pulmonary Edema

Initial treatment of acute cardiogenic pulmonary edema consists of oxygen, intravenous diuretic drugs, sublingual nitroglycerin, and morphine. Intubation with mechanical ventilation may be necessary for patients with progressive respiratory insufficiency despite these measures.

☑ *Severe pulmonary edema may require urgent intubation.*

Indications for Pulmonary Artery Balloon Flotation Catheter (Swan-Ganz)

Patients with acute cardiogenic pulmonary edema generally do not require a pulmonary artery catheter. However, catheter insertion may be useful in those not responding appropriately to therapy or those in whom it is unclear whether the pulmonary edema is due to cardiac versus non-cardiac causes.

Placement of a pulmonary artery catheter is more commonly useful in patients with cardiogenic shock unless there is rapid response to fluid administration (see pages 229–230).

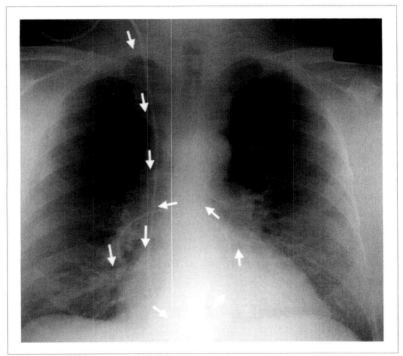

Figure 11-3. *Pathway for a Swan-Ganz catheter.*

"Why I like the right IJ approach for Swan-Ganz catheter placement..."

Placement of a Swan-Ganz catheter is an important skill in the patient with decompensated heart failure. It should be done reliably, safely, economically, and with minimal patient discomfort. Placing a venous sheath in the right internal jugular vein allows a straight access to the right atrium and right ventricle where a balloon tip catheter will make a natural curve into the pulmonary artery in most cases.

Complications from this site are uncommon; the most frequent in my experience is entry into the carotid artery. This usually occurs with a small diameter "finding" needle used to anesthetize the area. Adverse sequelae from carotid artery entry are rare. Pneumothorax is much less common with a right internal jugular approach than with the subclavian vein.

Position a patient as comfortably as possible, usually in a slight head down Trendelenberg position unless the patient is short of breath. I prep the right side of the neck and upper chest with Betadine, but do not lay a drape across their face until I have finished preparing. I remove the patient's pillow just prior to beginning the actual administration of local anesthetic. I prefer a thin 27 gauge by 4 cm needle to find the right jugular vein followed by a short (4 cm) 18 gauge thin wall needle on a 3 cc syringe to enter the vein after it is located.

I locate the right internal jugular vein by starting between the two heads of the sternocleidomastoid muscle, typically three finger breadths left of the patient's suprasternal notch and three finger breadths above the clavicle. I will often seek the vein by directing the anesthetizing needle slightly laterally and then marching medially. Once the anesthetizing needle has entered the internal jugular vein and blood return is obtained, I touch the 18 gauge thin wall needle to the patient's skin just prior to removal of the 27 gauge needle. Without delay, I gradually advance the 18 gauge thin wall needle into the right internal jugular vein until blood return is obtained. If the vein has seemingly "moved" after 2 or 3 passes, I apply local pressure briefly and again locate the vein with a small 25–27 gauge needle.

From the right internal jugular vein, the balloon tip catheter reliably advances into the right ventricle even in the presence of significant tricuspid regurgitation. At times, going from the right ventricle into the pulmonary artery is difficult. This usually occurs when the proximal catheter shaft prolapses into the inferior vena cava. In the absence of fluoroscopy, I often try to withdraw the catheter back into the right atrium and with a clockwise motion advance the catheter forward to achieve the pulmonary artery position. At times, I add a second milliliter of air into the balloon tip to facilitate this. Once pulmonary capillary wedge position is obtained, the balloon is deflated and the sheath is sutured in place.

Only rarely is fluoroscopy needed for advancement of the balloon tip catheter from the right internal jugular vein into the pulmonary artery.

The IJ approach provides a safe and effective method for Swan-Ganz placement.

Werner Forssmann

(1904-1979)

Werner Forssmann was the first to perform a catheterization of the right sided chambers of the heart in man and to publish his findings. His accomplishment is notable in that he performed this catheterization on himself.

Forssmann graduated from medical school at age 25. Later that year, after performing a series of procedures on cadavers, he advanced a urologic catheter from a cut-down on his left arm vein. A nurse held a mirror in front of an x-ray screen that allowed him to advance the catheter into his right atrium. He demonstrated that he was able to do this safely by walking up a set of stairs to have a chest x-ray film performed (Figure 11-5).[3]

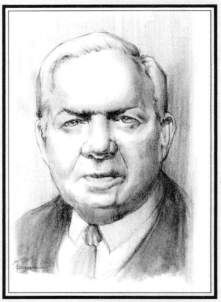

Figure 11-4. *Werner Forssmann.* Illustration by Peter Chapman.

Subsequently, he also performed simple angiographic contrast evaluations through a catheter including animal experiments using contrast media to visualize cardiac chambers.

Forssmann did not follow up on these initial clinical experiments but was recognized in 1956 by sharing the Nobel Prize in medicine with Drs. Andre Cournand and Dickinson Richards. Forssmann's insight and courage allowed him to test a new method that could be safely applied in a variety of clinical situations. In so doing, he anticipated subsequent developments in cardiac catheterization.

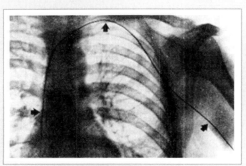

Figure 11-5. *Example of the catheter experiments performed by Werner Forssmann.*

Persistent Heart Failure

Treatment of either pulmonary or systemic congestion remains a central goal of therapy of acute heart failure. If patients have only been on moderate doses of diuretics as outpatients, you can increase doses or administer intravenous loop diuretics. For refractory volume overload, interventions such as continuous bumetanide (Bumex®, 0.25 to 2 mg per hour) infusion in addition to an oral thiazide-type diuretic such as metolazone may be useful. Continuous IV dopamine at a "renal range" of 1-3 µg/kg per minute is also a potent diuretic intervention. An increase in cardiac contractility likely contributes to renal vasodilatation at this dose. Both mechanisms improve renal perfusion and promote diuresis.

You can at least temporarily improve symptoms related to pleural effusions or ascites by performing either thoracentesis or paracentesis. Following this an intensification of medical therapy should follow to reduce the likelihood of recurrence. In refractory cases, effective removal of fluid can be achieved with use of veno-venous hemofiltration.[4]

☑ *Thoracentesis or paracentesis can complement diuresis of patients with severe volume overload.*

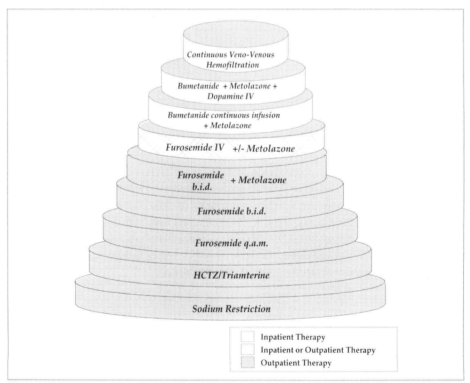

Figure 11-6. *Steps to treating persistent pulmonary or systemic congestion.*

Hemofiltration With or Without Dialysis

Hemofiltration with or without dialysis can allow the removal of 3-5 liters of fluid per day.[4] This requires placement of a two lumen central venous catheter (for example, Vascath®) and use of a special hemofiltration circuit in a properly supervised environment. Patients who may benefit from this include those who have acutely decompensated heart failure associated with profound systemic congestion in whom renal function is either acutely or chronically impaired. Depending on the type of filter that is used, removal of blood urea nitrogen and other waste products can be achieved in addition to removal of salt and water.

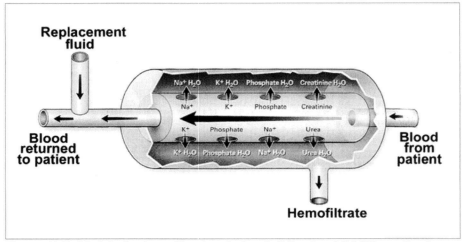

Figure 11-7. *Model of a hemofiltration device.* L.G.Forni and P.J.Hilton, Continuous hemofiltration in the treatment of acute renal failure. Vol. 336, 1304. Reprinted with permission from The New England Journal of Medicine, copyright © 1997 Massachusetts Medical Society. All rights reserved.[5]

Setting IV pump rates determines the amount of replacement fluid into the filter and hemofiltrate out from the filter. The difference in these two rates specifies the rate of fluid removed from the blood of the patient. In heart failure patients with refractory fluid retention associated with renal insufficiency — serum creatinine greater than 2.5 mg/dL — outpatient peritoneal dialysis may provide significant symptomatic improvement. This requires placement of a peritoneal Tenckhoff catheter under local anesthesia.[6]

Pharmacologic Management

In general, heart failure drugs have acute hemodynamic effects on vascular tone, ventricular contractility, or circulating vascular blood volume. Knowledge of these properties helps determine the suitability of a drug in an individual patient. Clinically, we assess a patient based on measurements of blood pressure and heart rate; history; physical exam; or laboratory estimates or measurements of cardiac output and filling pressures (see pages 18–21, 105–108). From these, first we infer a patient's initial circulatory physiology and second, predict physiologic effects of drug therapy.

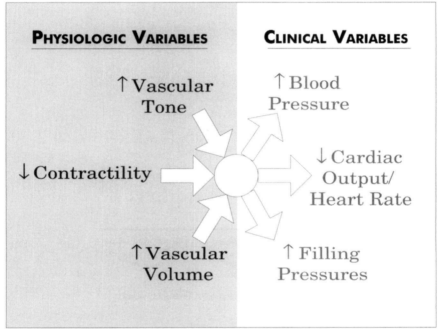

Figure 11-8. *Assessing the physiologic and clinical variables when managing heart failure.*

Intravenous Drug Therapy and Acute Heart Failure

Compared to a normal individual, the patient with compensated heart failure has a reduced reserve to circulatory stress including fluid overload, infection, ischemia, or arrhythmia. To treat a decompensated patient with worsening heart failure, short-term inotropic therapy is often beneficial. Drugs with positive myocardial inotropic effects are able to increase cardiac circulatory power beyond that of endogenous catecholamines alone. Recruiting additional myocardial reserve permits time to return a patient back to his state of compensated heart failure by avoiding a potential downhill spiral of progressive organ dysfunction and death. Nevertheless, if sustained for a long period of time, inotropic therapy may lead to adverse direct effects to the heart.

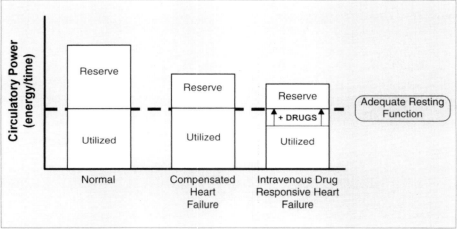

Figure 11-9. *Heart functioning circulatory power in energy/time.*

☑ *Commonly used intravenous medication for acute heart failure:*

- *Nitrates*
- *Milrinone*
- *Dobutamine*
- *Dopamine*

☑ *Consider use of milrinone in patients with decompensated heart failure on β-blockers.*

NITRATES (VASODILATORS)

Similar to oral nitrates, intravenous vasodilator therapy with nitroprusside or nitroglycerin can improve circulatory function by reducing preload and afterload without any direct effect on myocardial contractility. Nitrates act as precursors for nitric oxide also known as endothelium derived relaxing factor.

> **NITRATES**
> (Nitroprusside/Nitroglycerin)
> _____
> • Action mediated via nitric oxide
> • Increase intracellular c-GMP
> • Decrease intracellular Ca^{++}

☑ *Pharmacologic tolerance is greater with nitroglycerin than with nitroprusside.*

NITRIC OXIDE (VASODILATOR)

Nitric oxide is a neutral molecule with a free radical electron, making it highly reactive. Because of this reactivity, its biologic half-life is less than one minute. Nitric oxide can be administered as inhaled therapy for the treatment of increased pulmonary vascular resistance; however, this form of administration requires mechanical ventilation, advanced personnel training, and close supervision.

Use of either nitroprusside or nitroglycerin may lead to improvement in patients with acute heart failure.[7] Nitroprusside generates nitric oxide spontaneously whereas nitroglycerin requires free cell sulfhydryl groups in the endogenous chemical environment to do so. Although nitric oxide at high concentrations has negative myocardial inotropic effects, these effects are not seen with administration of intravenous nitrates. Nitric oxide activates a soluble guanylate cyclase which catalyses the formation of cyclic guanosine monophosphate (c-GMP) from guanosine triphosphate (GTP). Once formed, c-GMP acts as an intracellular secondary messenger to decrease intracellular calcium and vascular smooth muscle tone (see page 80).

NITRIC OXIDE

$$\cdot \overset{..}{N} = \overset{..}{\underset{..}{O}} :$$

Nitroprusside has a "balanced" action on dilating both arteries and veins. Nitroglycerin's action predominates on veins. Nevertheless, both lead to decreases in mean arterial and venous pressures.[8] Nitroglycerin is less likely to shunt blood flow from ischemic myocardium and may be preferable in acute myocardial ischemia syndromes such as heart failure with angina pectoris or myocardial infarction.[9]

☑ *IV therapy of heart failure affects inotropic state and vascular tone through changes in c-AMP and c-GMP.*

Milrinone (Inotrope/Vasodilator)

The phosphodiesterase inhibitor, milrinone, acts by increasing intracellular c-AMP in both heart and vascular muscle cells by blocking its breakdown. This combined mechanism of increased contractility and vasodilatation is effective at reducing elevated left and right heart filling pressures.[10] It is pharmacologically more potent than the older related drug, amrinone, and does not elicit the side effect of thrombocytopenia. Unlike other intravenous agents used in acute heart failure syndromes, milrinone has a biologic half-life of 2-3 hours. Because of this, milrinone requires a loading dose to have a rapid onset of action, and when stopped, it will persist for several hours within the circulation.

> **Milrinone (and Amrinone)**
>
> - Phosphodiesterase III inhibitors
> - Increase intracellular c-AMP in both heart and vascular muscle
> - Result in increased cardiac contractility and vasodilation

☑ *If needed, combining a phosphodiesterase inhibitor with a catecholamine can yield greater hemodynamic effects than either alone.*

Dobutamine (Inotrope)

Dobutamine is a potent, β_1-agonist resulting in increased myocyte c-AMP and cardiac contractility. It is also a moderate β_2-agonist resulting in modest vascular smooth muscle vasodilatation. Dobutamine is a racemic compund — existing as equal amounts of two optical isomers with the same chemical structure. One isomer acts as a mild α-agonist and the other acts as a mild α-antagonist. These two α effects tend to balance.[11] Thus dobutamine is a predominant positive inotrope medication. In an individual patient, however, its effects might be complex in part, depending on the pre-drug level of activation of the patient's α-receptors by endogenous sympathetic norepinephrine.

> **Dobutamine**
>
> - Potent β_1-agonist resulting in increased heart c-AMP
> - Mild β_2-agonist
> - Optically active 50:50 mixture of mild α-agonist and antagonist isomers

DOPAMINE (INOTROPE/VASOCONSTRICTOR)

Dopamine has multiple dose dependent mechanisms of action.[12] At low doses (< 3 μg/kg/min) it is effectively a diuretic via activation of dopaminergic receptors to increase renal blood flow. Dopamine at moderate doses (3-5 μg/kg/min), activates dopaminergic and β-adrenergic receptors and so is also a positive inotrope. At higher doses, dopamine acts as an arterial and venous vasoconstrictor. It is said that dopamine at high doses (> 5 μg/kg/min) is like norepinephrine (Levophed®). Dopamine does so because as the immediate precursor to norepinephrine within vesicles of sympathetic nerve terminals, it releases preformed stores of norepinephrine.[13] This is called a "tyramine" like effect. Thus, at high doses dopamine isn't just like norepinephrine, it *is* norepinephrine. Since patients with heart failure may have depleted endogenous stores of norepinephrine, if a patient has hypotension refractory to 10 μg/kg/min or higher of dopamine, I add norepinephrine directly instead of even higher doses of dopamine.

In cases of profound hemodynamic collapse with hypotension, use of boluses of epinephrine can help resuscitate a patient.

DOPAMINE

- Dopaminergic and β-agonist at low to moderate doses
- α-agonist at high dose (>5 μg/kg/min) secondary to tyramine like effect to release endogenous pre-synaptic NE

☑ *Dopamine is most commonly used to increase blood pressure or urine output.*

☑ *Dopamine at high doses releases endogenous norepinephrine.*

Comparative Hemodynamic Effects of Nitroprusside vs. Milrinone

In a group of eleven patients with New York Heart Association, Class III and IV heart failure, we compared a range of doses of nitroprusside to a range of doses of milrinone.[10] By matching the doses of each drug that led to the same fall in mean aortic pressure, we were able to assess the effects of the positive inotropic actions of milrinone beyond that due to decreased afterload alone.

Measurements were made during infusions in the cardiac catheterization lab. With nitroprusside, no effect was seen on contractility as measured by left ventricular peak rate of rise of pressure during isovolumic systole — Peak +dP/dt. Despite lack of direct cardiac effect with nitroprusside, stroke work rose as left ventricular end- diastolic pressure fell.

$$\text{STROKE WORK} = \text{STROKE VOLUME X (MEAN ARTERIAL PRESSURE -} \text{LEFT VENTRICULAR FILLING PRESSURE)}$$

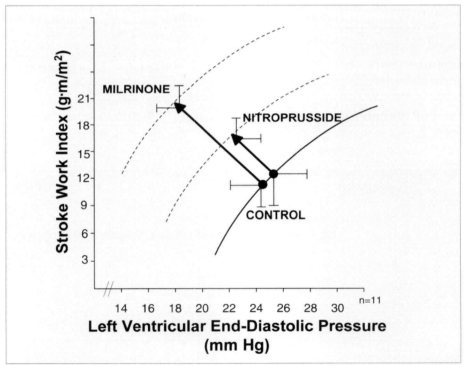

Figure 11-10. *Effects of nitroprusside and milrinone on LV performance at matched mean aortic pressure.*[10]

☑ *For a similar decrease in mean aortic pressure, milrinone led to a greater decrease in left heart filling pressure.*

With milrinone, at *matched mean aortic pressure*, left ventricluar Peak +dP/dt increased associated with a greater increase in stroke work index and a greater fall in left ventricular filling pressure. Thus, for any decrease in mean aortic pressure, the inotropic effects of milrinone led to measurable greater improvements in ventricular function and falls in filling pressure.

Alternatively, when doses of nitroprusside and milrinone were compared that gave the same increase *in cardiac index* (approximately 50%), the fall in left heart filling pressures were similar. With this matched cardiac index comparison, however, mean arterial pressure decreased approximately twice as much with nitroprusside as with milrinone. Thus, inotropic stimulation of the heart with milrinone blunts decreases in mean arterial pressure associated with vasodilator effects alone. This may be important since pure vasodilator therapy alone is ultimately limited by hypotension.

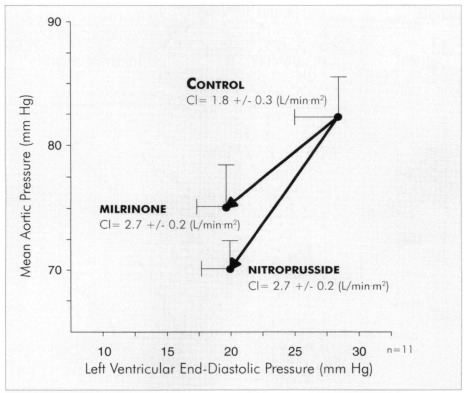

Figure 11-11. *An inotrope vasodilator (milrinone) can improve cardiac performance with preservation of aortic pressure compared to pure vasodilator (nitroprusside) therapy alone.*[10]

Comparative Hemodynamic Effects of Milrinone vs. Dobutamine

In a group of 15 patients with NYHA Class III and IV heart failure, we gave a range of 2 to 14 µg/kg/min of dobutamine and compared it to a range of doses of milrinone.[14] Heart rate went up moderately with both drugs. Left ventricular filling pressure (measured in the cardiac catheterization lab directly as left ventricular end-diastolic pressure) fell modestly with dobutamine, but more with milrinone (dobutamine −29%; milrinone −46%). Mean arterial pressure was unchanged with dobutamine, but it decreased about 10 mm Hg with milrinone. Cardiac index showed a trend to increase more with milrinone.

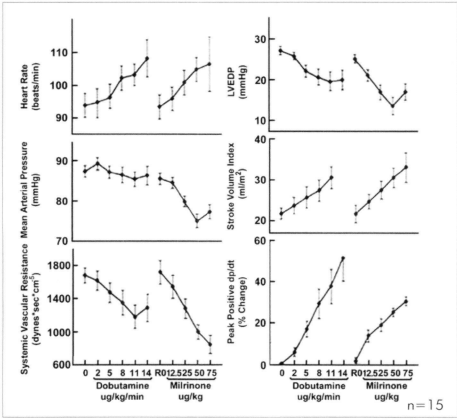

Figure 11-12. *At high doses, dobutamine led to greater increases in contractility. Milrinone led to greater decreases in left ventricular filling pressure and afterload.* Reproduced with permission. (Colucci WS, Wright RF, Jaski BE, Fifer MA, Braunwald E. Milrinone and dobutamine in severe heart failure: differing hemodynamic effects and individual patient responsiveness. Circulation 1986; 73:III177).[14]

Systemic vascular resistance fell more with milrinone (dobutamine –29%; milrinone –51%). Peak rate of left ventricular pressure increase during isovolumic systole (Peak +dP/dt) increased with both drugs but more with dobutamine (dobutamine +50%; milrinone +30%). At high doses then, dobutamine is a more potent inotrope and milrinone is a more potent vasodilator.

Comparison of Dobutamine vs. Dopamine

Both dobutamine and dopamine increase cardiac output. At 10 µg/kg/min, dopamine's inotropic and vasoconstrictor effects will lead to an increase in blood pressure. At this dose, filling pressure *increases* with dopamine due to an increase in ventricular afterload and venous tone.[15]

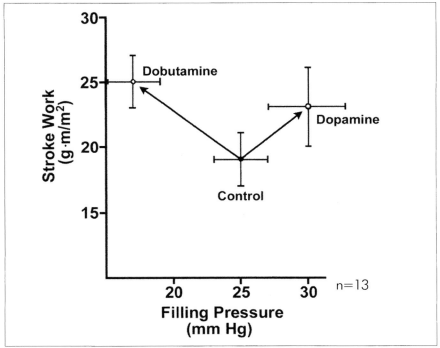

Figure 11-13. *Frank-Starling curve of dobutamine vs. dopamine: Effect on stroke work versus filling pressure at 10µg/kg/min. At high doses, dobutamine and dopamine lead to opposite effects on left heart filling pressure.* Reproduced with permission.(Loeb HS, Bredakis J, Gunner RM. Superiority of dobutamine over dopamine for augmentation of cardiac output in patients with chronic low output cardiac failure. Circulation 1977; 55:378).[15]

Dobutamine, Milrinone, and Nitroprusside: Effects on LV Contractility vs. Afterload

Figure 11-14 summarizes changes in contractility (shown on the vertical axis as the percent change in $+dP/dt$) versus afterload (shown on the horizontal axis as percent change in systemic vascular resistance) seen with nitroprusside, milrinone, and dobutamine.[14] Nitroprusside has no effect on contractility but is a potent vasodilator. Milrinone leads to the greatest fall in calculated systemic vascular resistance with an intermediate effect on increasing myocardial contractility. Finally, dobutamine has the greatest effect on contractility at high doses with some vasodilator properties.

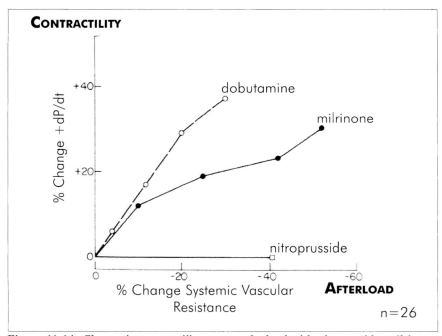

Figure 11-14. *Change in contractility versus afterload with nitropruside, milrinone, and dobutamine.* Reproduced with permission. (Colucci WS, Wright RF, Jaski BE, Fifer MA, Braunwald E. Milrinone and dobutamine in severe heart failure: differing hemodynamic effects and individual patient responsiveness. Circulation 1986; 73:III178).[14]

☑ *Milrinone's effects are similar to the combination of dobutamine and nitroprusside.*

Summary of Hemodynamic Effects of Intravenous Therapy

The effects of vasoactive intravenous agents are depicted in Figure 11-15 — a plot of *contractility* on the vertical axis and *vascular tone* on the horizontal axis. In general, agents that decrease vascular tone or increase contractility, increase cardiac output. Pure vasodilators that decrease vascular tone also lead to a decrease in blood pressure. Conversely, agents that are vasoconstrictors and that increase vascular tone increase blood pressure. All are catecholamines except milrinone and the nitrates. In acute decompensated heart failure, agents that decrease contractility are avoided.

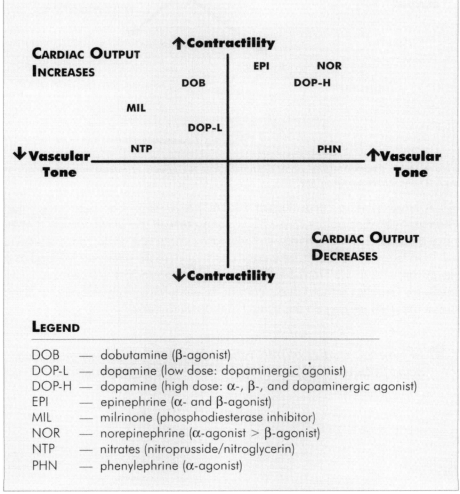

Figure 11-15. *Intravenous medications and their impact on hemodynamics.*

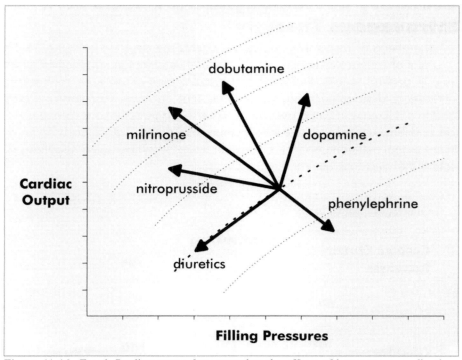

Figure 11-16. *Frank-Starling curve demonstrating the effects of intravenous medications on left ventricular performance.*

A Frank-Starling curve (Figure 11-16) presentation can depict expected changes in cardiac output versus filling pressures with use of vasoactive intravenous medications. Medications that increase contractility or decrease afterload will lead to an upward shift, whereas those that increase afterload will lead to a downward shift in the Frank-Starling curve. Vasoconstrictors will increase filling pressure. Diuretics without direct cardiac or vascular actions will reduce filling pressures while staying on the same Frank-Starling curve.

☑ *In general, studies of intravenous medication in decompensated heart failure come from patients with systolic dysfunction.*

Effects of Nitroprusside, Milrinone, and Dobutamine on Global Myocardial Oxygen Consumption

The effects of vasoactive medications go beyond hemodynamics alone.[16] Effects on myocardial oxygen consumption may be relevant to heart failure drug selection when you are concerned about myocardial ischemia. This comparison (Figure 11-17) shows the effects of nitroprusside, milrinone, and dobutamine on myocardial oxygen consumption in ten heart failure patients studied in the cardiac catheterization lab. The nitrate, nitroprusside, led to a decrease in myocardial oxygen consumption. There was no net change with the phosphodiesterase inhibitor, milrinone. There was an increase with dobutamine.

Nitrates may decrease myocardial oxygen consumption by decreasing afterload through a decrease in arterial pressure and a decrease in left ventricular size through the LaPlace relationship.

Milrinone will have effects on myocardial oxygen consumption as a vasodilator (similar to nitrates) offset by effects on increases in contractility. Dobutamine will increase contractility and lead to a moderate increase in myocardial oxygen consumption.

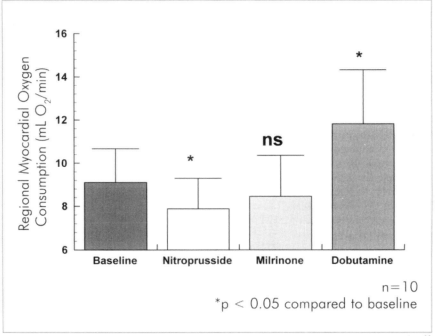

Figure 11-17. *The effects of intravenous medications on myocardial oxygen consumption.*[16]

Dopamine vs. Dobutamine

Because of dopamine's effects on increasing arterial and ventricular filling pressures, dopamine will lead to an increase in myocardial oxygen consumption greater than that of dobutamine.[17] Figure 11-18 shows the effect of dopamine on an indirect measure of myocardial oxygen consumption — the product of heart rate and systolic blood pressure — over a range of doses. Dopamine led to a greater increase in this index of myocardial oxygen consumption than achieved with dobutamine, despite a greater increase in cardiac index with dobutamine. Associated with this was a greater increase in premature ventricular contractions seen with dopamine compared with dobutamine (Figure 11-19).

Figure 11-18. *The impact of dopamine and dobutamine on myocardial oxygen consumption.* Reproduced with permission. (Leier CV, Heban PT, Huss P, Bush CA, Lewis RP. Comparative systemic and regional hemodynamic effects of dopamine and dobutamine in patients with cardiomyopathic heart failure. Circulation 1978; 58:473).[17]

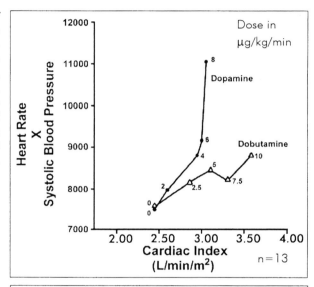

Figure 11-19. *Premature ventricular contractions associated with dopamine and dobutamine.* Reproduced with permission. (Leier CV, Heban PT, Huss P, Bush CA, Lewis RP. Comparative systemic and regional hemodynamic effects of dopamine and dobutamine in patients with cardiomyopathic heart failure. Circulation 1978; 58:473).[17]

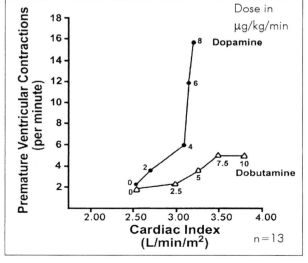

Approach to the Intravenous Therapy of the Acute Heart Failure Patient: The Hemodynamic Diagram

My approach to intravenous pharmacologic therapy in patients with decompensated heart failure and left ventricular systolic dysfunction is summarized in Figure 11-20. On the vertical axis is an index of afterload that is easily obtained — systolic blood pressure. On the horizontal axis is an estimate of a patient's left ventricular preload shown as pulmonary capillary wedge pressure (PCW). This wedge pressure does not need to be measured with a Swan-Ganz catheter if it can be estimated based on clinical criteria. For example, if a patient has pulmonary edema, it is likely that the wedge pressure is high. Conversely, if a patient has had a gastrointestinal syndrome with nausea, vomiting, or diarrhea and has poor skin turgor consistent with intravascular depletion, it is likely that the wedge pressure is low. In other cases, however, you may need to measure a wedge pressure with a pulmonary artery floatation catheter to optimally approach the treatment of your decompensated heart failure patient.

If a patient is volume depleted, then a volume challenge of either normal saline or a colloid, such as Plasmanate®, should be given prior to drug infusion. An adequate filling pressure is likely present when pulmonary wedge pressure is 18 mm Hg or higher. This may need to

☑ *If the patient is "dry," give volume before drugs.*

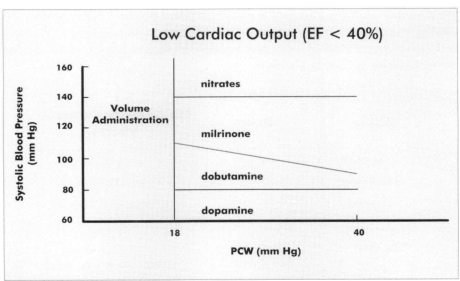

Figure 11-20. *Hemodynamic diagram for the acute heart failure patient.*

☑ *You may clinically estimate or directly measure wedge pressure via a Swan-Ganz catheter.*

be higher in intubated patients receiving positive end-expiratory pressure.

When filling pressure is adequate or high and a patient is still in a low cardiac output state, my choice of drug relates to the systolic blood pressure. If blood pressure is high, then a pure vasodilator such as nitroprusside or nitroglycerin can lead to significant improvements in cardiac index and lower filling pressures. If the blood pressure is lower, particularly in the face of marked pulmonary edema, then a phosphodiesterase inhibitor, milrinone, should lead to more rapid clinical improvement. If blood pressure is at a borderline level then dobutamine may be a better drug as mean arterial pressure will, in general, not change with this, but modest decreases in left ventricular filling pressure will still result.

☑ *Milrinone is useful in rapidly reversing acute pulmonary edema.*

Finally, if a patient is hypotensive with a systolic blood pressure of less than 80 mm Hg, then the combined α- and β-agonist effects of dopamine will allow improvement of blood pressure while, hopefully, a reversible etiology of decompensated heart failure is identified and treated. When this is not possible, mechanical support devices may be appropriate, such as an intra-aortic balloon pump.

As you move down this ladder of medications (Figure 11-21), therapy changes from drugs that decrease myocardial oxygen consumption with the nitrates, to no change in myocardial oxygen consumption with phosphodiesterase inhibitors, to progressive increases in myocardial oxygen consumption with catecholamines. In susceptible patients, higher myocardial oxygen consumption may lead to greater risk for myocardial ischemia or arrhythmia. Nevertheless, the drug that promptly improves a decompensated patient's hemodynamics is usually the best since improvement will be associated with a reduction of potent endogenous mediators of increased myocardial oxygen consumption such as norepinephrine and epinephrine.

Agent	Dose	Major Hemodynamic Effects
nitroprusside	10-400 µg/min	Vasodilation
nitroglycerin	10-400 µg/min	Vasodilation
milrinone	50 µg/kg over 10 min 0.25-0.75 µg/kg/min	Inotrope, Vasodilation
dobutamine	2-14 µg/kg/min	Inotrope
dopamine	1-3 µg/kg/min	Vasodilation
	3-10 µg/kg/min	Inotrope, Vasoconstriction
norepinephrine	0.5-5 µg/min	Inotrope, Vasoconstriction
phenylephrine	10-100 µg/min	Vasoconstriction

Figure 11-21. *Doses of IV medications.*

Limitations of IV Agents

Although vasoactive intravenous medications can be helpful in decompensated heart failure, no one drug is a panacea. All are often used in combination with a diuretic. Because any drug may have variable effects in a given patient, initially it is best to use a single vasoactive agent that is likely to improve a patient's condition rather than multiple drugs at the outset. Recent studies with intravenous human B-type natriuretic peptide (hBNP) suggest that this may be a useful additional agent in the future.[18]

Class	Agent	Limitation
Nitrates	nitroprusside	Hypotension
	nitroglycerin	Tolerance (NTG>NTP)
Phosphodiesterase Inhibitors	milrinone	Slow offset of action
	amrinone	Slow offset of action, Thrombocytopenia
Catecholamines	dobutamine	Tolerance (β-receptor down regulation)
	dopamine	Tolerance, Central venous access used

In general, intravenous medications are used only as long as necessary to maintain hemodynamic stability while precipitating factors are identified and treated. Once this has been achieved, intravenous therapy should be weaned and substituted for chronic oral therapy.

CHRONIC USE OF INTRAVENOUS INOTROPES

Long-term continuous administration of dobutamine or milrinone may serve as an "intravenous inotropic bridge" to cardiac transplantation. In refractory patients who are not candidates for cardiac transplant, intermittent or continuous intravenous inotropic therapy for chronic heart failure may permit hospital discharge.[19] Although acute symptoms may improve, the effects of this therapy on morbidity and mortality are uncertain (see page 43). Patients receiving continuous home inotropic therapy should have adequate social support and home health follow-up. Placement of an indwelling central venous catheter (Groshong or Hickman) with use of a portable pump facilitates patient mobility.

Acute Myocardial Infarction and Heart Failure

Patients with acute heart failure and evidence of acute myocardial injury/ infarction should be considered for urgent cardiac catheterization. Depending on the anatomic extent of coronary artery disease, revascularization of the infarct related artery via balloon angioplasty or intracoronary stenting has a technical success rate up to 98%.[20-22] Consider intravenous thrombolysis with t-PA, reteplase, or streptokinase if these procedures cannot be done expeditiously.

When patients with an acute myocardial infarction develop heart failure, the 12-lead ECG can help you determine which mechanical syndromes are likely contributing etiologies (Figure 11-22). In inferior myocardial infarction, the presence of right ventricular infarction implies a proximal right coronary artery occlusion. Findings of hypotension, neck vein distention and clear lung fields associated with ST elevation in the right-sided ECG lead V4R support this. Acute mitral regurgitation due to left ventricular posterior papillary muscle ischemia can follow an occlusion of a right dominant coronary artery.[23]

Conversely with Q-waves and elevation of anterior ST segments (leads V1-2-3), heart failure is more commonly related to a left anterior descending coronary artery occlusion with extensive infarction, ventricular aneurysm, or ventricular septal defect formation. Cardiac rupture with tamponade and acute cardiovascular collapse may accompany either inferior or anterior myocardial infarction.

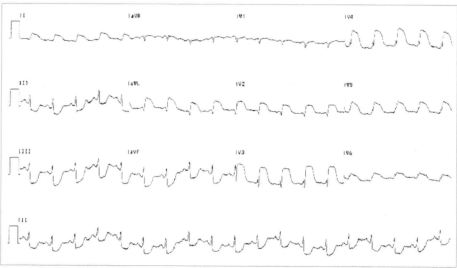

Figure 11-22. *ECG showing acute anterior MI in a patient with heart failure.*

SPECIFIC HEART FAILURE SYNDROMES WITH Q-WAVE INFARCTION[23]

MI Location	Coronary Artery Occlusion	Q-waves	Syndromes
Inferior	Right	Leads II, III, AVF	Right ventricular infarction with high venous pressure low output Acute mitral regurgitation due to posterior papillary muscle ischemia
Anterior	Left Anterior Descending (LAD)	Leads V1-2-3	Cardiogenic shock due to extensive infarction Ventricular aneurysm Septal rupture

☑ *The ECG helps identify heart failure syndromes in acute MI.*

Cardiogenic Shock

CARDIOGENIC SHOCK

Heart failure with severe systemic hypoperfusion usually with hypotension and pulmonary edema.

Patients who develop cardiogenic shock present dramatically. Their skin is cold and clammy; mental status may be abnormal; breathing is labored. Patients are more likely weak than agitated as in pulmonary edema without shock.

The most common cause of cardiogenic shock is acute myocardial infarction. When 40% or more of the left ventricle is involved with either previous or acute myocardial infarction cardiogenic shock will usually follow.[24] Following acute myocardial infarction, cardiogenic shock may not initially be present but can develop over the following 24-hours. In patients receiving thrombolysis who manifest cardiogenic shock during their hospitalization, only 15% had overt cardiogenic shock at the time of admission (GUSTO I trial).[25] Goldberg and coworkers, in an observational community study, found that the incidence of cardiogenic shock with acute myocardial infarction remained relatively stable between 1975 and 1997 at an average of 7.1%. Although the overall mortality following cardiogenic shock was 71.7%, there was a trend toward a decreased in-hospital mortality in the mid- to late-1990's associated with a greater use of coronary reperfusion strategies.[26]

DRUG TREATMENT OF CARDIOGENIC SHOCK

If unresponsive to fluid administration, cardiogenic shock requires inotropic intravenous therapy. Administer dopamine, dobutamine, or milrinone based on a patient's presentation with hypotension and/or pulmonary edema (see page 227). Respiratory failure should lead to intubation and mechanical ventilation.

☑ *If necessary, 0.1 – 1.0 mg boluses of IV epinephrine can temporarily maintain the circulation until mechanical support can be initiated.*

INTRA-AORTIC BALLOON PUMP (IABP)

Intra-aortic balloon counterpulsation may be indicated in patients, especially in the setting of urgent coronary artery revascularization for acute myocardial injury/infarction. In the setting of acute MI and cardiogenic shock, IABP on average will increase cardiac output 0.5 L/min (see pages 235–241). Total circulatory support with percutaneous extracorporeal life support (ECLS) is an option for the patient refractory to intra-aortic balloon pump undergoing percutaneous revascularization in the cardiac catheterization lab (see pages 243–246).[27]

☑ *Intra-aortic balloon pump may also be used for cases of non-coronary cardiogenic shock such as myocarditis or heart transplant rejection.[28]*

THE SHOCK TRIAL

The SHOCK (Should We Emergently Revascularize Occluded Coronaries for Cardiogenic Shock) trial compared early revascularization to initial medical stabilization in 302 patients with acute myocardial infarction and cardiogenic shock. Early revascularization showed a trend to a better outcome in the primary endpoint 30-day mortality at 46.7% vs. 56.0%, p<0.09. The median time from the onset of infarction to shock was 5.6 hours. In the revascularization group, 32.7% had sustained a cardiac arrest and 86.2% had intra-aortic balloon placement. Out of the group of patients assigned to early revascularization 86.8% were able to undergo either angioplasty or bypass surgery. Because of a high incidence of left main and three vessel coronary artery disease patients in this trial, 36% underwent initial bypass surgery without attempted angioplasty. During angioplasty, 74% of patients underwent stent placement in the most recent 1997-98 subgroup.[29]

Initial Treatment of Sudden Death: Advanced Cardiac Life Support (ACLS)

In a pulseless patient, advanced cardiac life support algorithms are appropriate.[30] Either ventricular tachycardia or ventricular fibrillation should be treated with prompt defibrillation. Consider use of IV amiodarone for recurrent monomorphic ventricular tachycardia (see page 187). When a patient has recurrent polymorphic ventricular tachycardia — changing morphology of the wide complex beats or Torsades de Pointes — consider that this may be a drug or electrolyte abnormality associated with a long QT interval. Acutely, this may respond to magnesium or lidocaine. If bradycardia is present, ventricular pacing may be necessary to shorten the prolonged QT interval for recurrent arrhythmia. Drugs that lengthen the QT interval such as procainamide should, in general, be avoided.

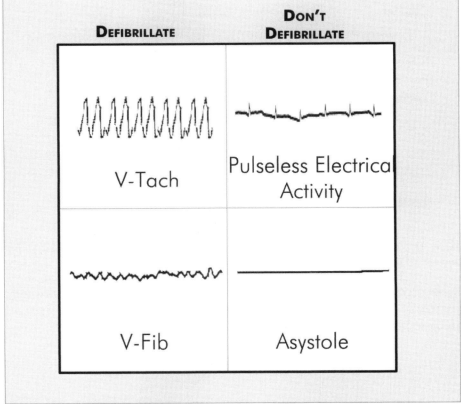

Figure 11-23. *Defibrillation is appropriate when a patient is in V-Tach or V-Fib.*

☑ *In a patient with recurrent ventricular tachycardia consider the diagnosis of Torsades de Pointes.*

Treatment of pulseless electrical activity (also called electrical-mechanical dissociation) requires identification of the cause. It is important to consider pericardial tamponade as a possible etiology, as immediate pericardiocentesis can be life saving. Any cause of electrical-mechanical dissociation may initially respond to intravenous epinephrine. Finally, electrical asystole may be due to marked metabolic derangements or follow prolonged cardiovascular collapse of any cause.

Symptom	Etiology	Treatment
V-Tach	Myocardial ischemia	Defibrillate
	Electrolyte abnormality	Amiodarone
V-Fib	Myocardial ischemia	Defibrillate
	Electrolyte abnormality	Amiodarone
Pulseless Electrical Activity	Massive pulmonary embolism	Thrombolysis, surgical embolectomy
	Pericardial tamponade	Pericardiocentesis
	Aortic dissection	Surgery
	Massive hemmorhage	Transfusion, surgery
	Profound LV dysfunction	Mechanical support
Asystole	Metabolic Late finding of above	Epinephrine

Figure 11-24. *Symptoms, etiologies, and treatments of conditions requiring advanced life support.*

In a patient with end-stage heart failure who is not a candidate for cardiac transplant, discussion of a "do not attempt" resuscitation status with a patient and family is appropriate prior to acute decompensation.

Mechanical Circulatory Assist

When acute heart failure results in hemodynamic compromise, endogenous or exogenous inotropic stimulation can improve heart function, but at the potential cost of myocardial ischemia. Mechanical assist devices supplement myocardial biochemical reserve with hydraulic energy derived from external sources. Mechanical assistance increases total circulatory resting power to allow:

    1). The maintenance of adequate circulatory function

    2). A decrease in utilized cardiac function

    3). An increase in reserve function

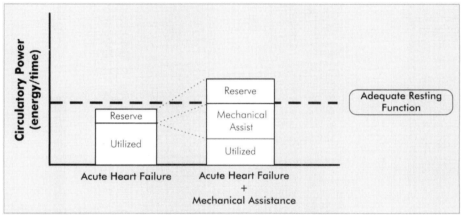

Figure 11-25. *Hemodynamics of mechanical circulatory assistance.*

The Pathway from Stabilization to Intervention

The need for mechanical circulatory assistance is based on the etiology of cardiac failure as well as the pace of hemodynamic deterioration (Figure 11-26). Initial treatment is with conventional intravenous therapy or with advanced cardiac life support (ACLS) protocol.[30]

Intravascular depletion should be considered initially in any patient. Myocardial ischemia and ventricular arrhythmias may occur when greater inotropic stimulation is necessary to maintain adequate circulatory flow and arterial pressure.

In heart failure associated with acute myocardial ischemia, mechanical assistance or supported coronary revascularization may allow salvage of myocardium. Hemodynamic stabilization can permit diagnostic and therapeutic procedures to be performed more safely.

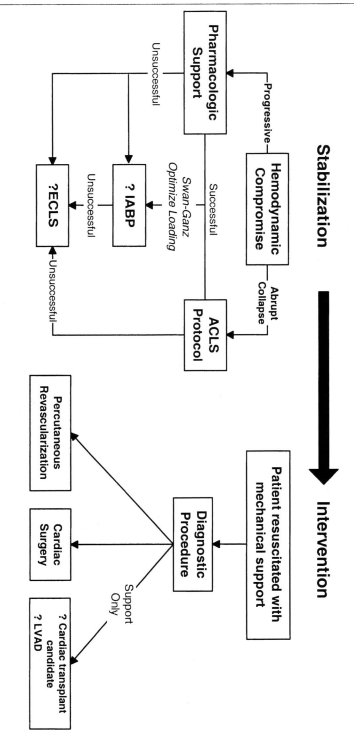

Figure 11-26. *Heart failure and mechanical support.* Adapted from Jaski BE, Branch KR. Supported circulation in the cardiac catheterization laboratory. In: Peterson KL, Nicod P, editors. Cardiac catheterization: Methods, diagnosis, and therapy. 1997:549.[31] By permission of the publisher, WB Saunders Company Limited.

ACLS — Advanced cardiac life support
IABP — Intra-aortic balloon pump
ECLS — Percutaneous extracorporeal life support
LVAD — Left ventricular assist device

Intra-aortic Balloon Pump

INTRA-AORTIC BALLOON PUMP

An intravascular balloon that is inflated and deflated in the descending thoracic aorta from a percutaneous catheter in the femoral artery that supports the systemic and coronary circulations.

Timing of inflation and deflation of an intra-aortic balloon pump is critical for optimal hemodynamic effect. Intra-aortic balloon inflation should coincide with the closure of the aortic valve. Deflation should occur just prior to left ventricular ejection and aortic valve opening. Optimal placement of the intra-aortic balloon pump includes placing the balloon catheter tip just distal to the origin of the left subclavian artery in the descending thoracic aorta.

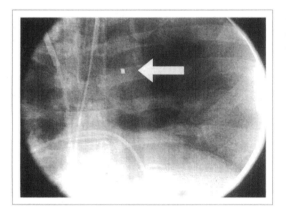

Figure 11-27. *X-ray image of a chest during IABP support. Arrow indicates distal tip of IABP catheter.*

TECHNIQUE FOR IABP INSERTION

1. Percutaneous access into femoral artery.
2. Insert J-type 0.032-0.038 inch guide wire into abdominal aorta. Place 8-French dilator and exchange for 11.5-12.5-French introducer sheath over wire.
3. Insert balloon leading with J-type 0.032 wire. If using fluoroscopic guidance, advance balloon and wire to aorta, just distal to origin of left subclavian artery from x-ray silhouette of thoracic aorta. Estimate this if no fluoroscopy available.
4. Administer heparin. Start balloon counterpulsation.

Mechanics of IABP Support

During balloon pump support, diastolic blood pressure typically exceeds systolic blood pressure.[31] Timed with cardiac diastole, intra-aortic balloon pump (IABP) inflation displaces blood volume within the aorta to increase total systemic and myocardial blood flow. Increased coronary perfusion pressure during diastole improves myocardial oxygen delivery when coronary vascular impedance to flow is low. Deflation of the balloon during cardiac systole reduces aortic volume and, therefore, decreases left ventricular afterload and myocardial oxygen consumption.

Figure 11-28. *Mechanics of IABP support.* Reprinted with permission. Quaal S, editor. Comprehensive intra-aortic balloon counterpulsation. St. Louis: Mosby, 1993:99.[32]

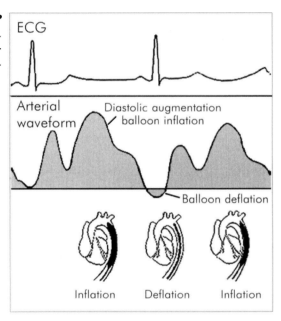

☑ *Aortic diastolic pressure should exceed systolic pressure during IABP support.*

☑ *Effects of IABP on Hemodynamics*

↓ SBP	↓ Myocardial O_2 demand
↑ DBP	↑ Myocardial blood flow
↑ Cardiac output	↓ Myocardial lactate production
↓ PCW	

IABP Effects on Myocardial Oxygen Demand vs. Perfusion

In patients with cardiogenic shock, IABP counterpulsation decreases systolic tension-time index (TTI), a measure of myocardial oxygen consumption. IABP augments diastolic pressure-time index (DPTI), an index of the coronary perfusion gradient (DPTI–LVDP). A decrease in myocardial oxygen consumption and an increase in coronary perfusion can improve left ventricular dysfunction associated with myocardial ischemia.[33-35]

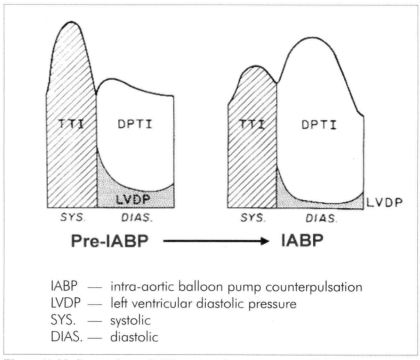

Figure 11-29. *Pre- and post- IABP support decreases myocardial oxygen consumption and increases coronary perfusion.* From Amsterdam EA, Awan NA, Lee G, et al: Intra-aortic balloon counterpulsation: Rationale, application, and results. In: Rackley CE [ed]: Critical Care Cardiology. Philadelphia, FA Davis, 1981 with permission of the publisher.[36,31]

Timing of Inflation and Deflation

Adjustment of the IABP to inflate throughout cardiac diastole (counterpulsation) is important to obtain maximal hemodynamic benefit.[32] The console initiates inflation by an operator or electronically determined interval after the occurrence of the ECG R-wave or arterial pressure peak. Depending on the type of console, deflation can either occur at the onset of the next R-wave (real timing) or following a set time interval after the onset of balloon inflation (conventional timing). Since the interval between electrical (QRS complex) and mechanical events (e.g. aortic valve opening) varies little with changes in heart rate or rhythm, newer designs utilize real timing to set deflation and inflation independent of heart rate or operator manipulation.

Real timing may also operate effectively with irregular cardiac rhythms having an identifiable R-wave — such as atrial fibrillation and premature ventricular contractions.[37] Real timing, however, can be limited by the ability of the console to evacuate the balloon gas prior to aortic ejection to prevent balloon obstruction to aortic outflow.

Indications for IABP

In general, patients on inotropes with clinical low-output syndrome despite adequate or elevated filling pressures and a low arterial pressure may benefit from IABP support.[32,38–40] During acute myocardial infarction, IABP placement may allow patient stability when the ejection fraction is less than 30% especially when treatment includes primary or post-thrombolytic PTCA. Ventricular failure associated with acute myocarditis may be refractory to pharmacologic therapy, but improve with IABP placement.[41] Active myocarditis or any acute onset of non-coronary shock treated with circulatory mechanical support including IABP can lead to ventricular recovery and avoid the need for urgent cardiac transplant.[28]

INDICATIONS FOR IABP AND HEART FAILURE

- Cardiogenic shock despite inotropic therapy
- Acute myocardial infarction complicated by mitral regurgitation or ventricular septal defect
- Acute myocarditis associated with shock
- Bridge to transplant

☑ *IABP may provide support for either ischemic or non-ischemic heart failure.*

CONTRAINDICATIONS AND COMPLICATIONS

Significant aortic aneurysms and dissections are at least relative contraindications to IABP placement due to an increased risk of aortic rupture. Marked aortic valve regurgitation is also a contraindication since increased diastolic pressure during balloon inflation will increase regurgitation into the left ventricle.

Peripheral vascular disease is a relative contraindication as catheter insertion may be impossible or associated with leg ischemia. Calcified arterial lesions may damage the integrity of the balloon causing it to fail during support, or the large sheath size may inhibit distal blood flow to the leg. Complications of peripheral vascular morbidity and leg ischemia with percutaneous insertion range from 11% to 21%.[31,42] Thus, leg ischemia remains the primary complication of IABP support. Predictors of leg ischemia include known peripheral vascular disease, smoking, diabetes, and female sex (due to smaller leg vessel diameters). In patients at high risk for ischemia, performance of ileofemoral contrast angiography prior to IABP insertion may assist in the decision to initiate IABP therapy and may be used to guide insertion site selection and aortic wire placement.

CONTRAINDICATIONS TO IABP

- Aortic aneurysms or dissection
- Aortic valve regurgitation
- Obstructive peripheral vascular disease
- Inability to insert cannulas
- Wire may assist placement into aorta
- Little or no native cardiac output

Examples of IABP Waveforms

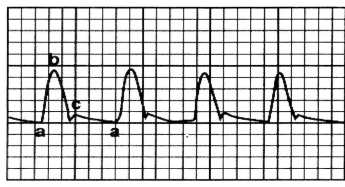

Figure 11-30. *Normal arterial waveform demonstrating: a – end-diastole; b – peak systole; c – dicrotic notch.*

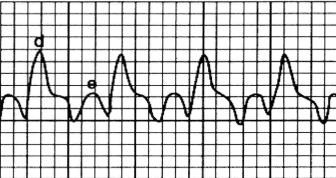

Figure 11-31. *IABP assisted arterial waveform demonstrating: d – peak diastolic augmentation; e – reduced systolic peak pressure.*

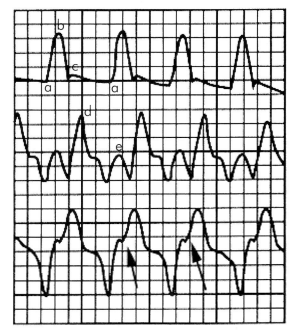

Figure 11-32. *Arterial pressure waveforms demonstrating unassisted, appropriately assisted, and inappropriate early inflation effect (arrows).*

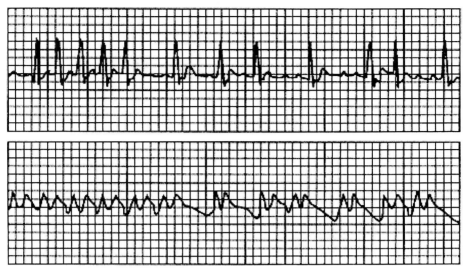

Figure 11-33. *Simultaneous ECG and aortic pressure tracing during irregular atrial flutter. IABP assist using real time timing responds accurately.*

John Gibbon
(1903-1979)

John Gibbon invented the first heart lung machine that completely assumed the circulatory and respiratory functions of the heart and lungs. This accomplishment provided the support for most subsequent cardiac surgery as well as the more recent application of resuscitation of patients following cardiovascular collapse.

After obtaining his M.D. degree, Gibbon began a research fellowship in surgery at Harvard Medical School when he was 27 years old. As an assistant, Gibbon cared for a woman with a massive pulmonary embolus by

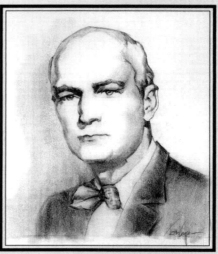

Figure 11-34. *John Gibbon.* Illustration by Peter Chapman

measuring her blood pressure every 15 minutes for a period of 17 hours. At that moment, he could no longer measure any blood pressure and an attempt was made to perform an operation to remove the blood clot in her pulmonary artery. The patient died despite this. During this ordeal, he thought about the value of a device that would remove blood from the veins, oxygenate it and return it back to the arterial system thus bypassing the blood clot in the pulmonary artery. Four years later, Gibbon developed a machine that was able to completely support the circulation and respiration of a cat after surgical closure of the main pulmonary artery. It was 18 years after this that the first successful patient operation was performed by Gibbon using his heart lung device, after many improvements, in an 18-year-old woman who had recurrent heart failure due to a large atrial septal defect. His successful use of extracorporeal life support was subsequently embraced by cardiac surgeons throughout the world.

Gibbon was remarkable for his persistence in achieving his goal. From an event that occurred during a clinical research experience, 20 years of overcoming innumerable technical and ethical obstacles resulted in his achieving a profound success.[43]

Percutaneous Extracorporeal Life Support (ECLS)

A *portable* extracorporeal life support system comprised of a pump, a heat exchanger, and an oxygenator is analogous in design to the heart-lung machine used during open-heart surgery.[44]

Deoxygenated blood flows from the venous circulation through a cannula and tubing to an external centrifugal blood pump mounted on the ECLS cart. Blood enters the apex of the pump where smooth surfaced, internal rotating cones transfer centrifugal energy to the blood to force it outward at increased speeds. The accelerated blood is allowed to "escape" at the widest part of the pump while blood is drawn in at the apex of the spinning cones to replace the expelled volume.

The accelerated blood passes through a heat exchanger where the blood is warmed to physiologic temperatures by circulating water, and an electromagnetic flow probe estimates total ECLS output. The blood then passes into a membrane oxygenator for gas exchange. Oxygen circulating through hollow fibers diffuses across a large membrane surface area and is exchanged for CO_2 in the passing blood. Blood exiting the membrane oxygenator circulates to the arterial cannula and is returned to the patient's arterial circulation.

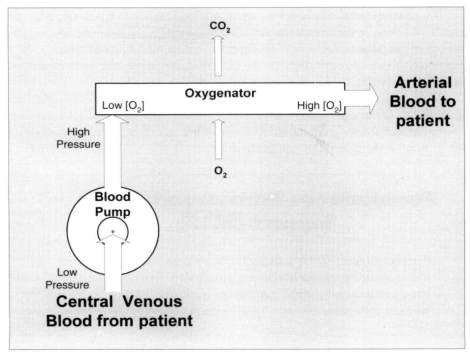

Figure 11-35. *Model of percutaneous ECLS.*

ECLS Catheters (Cannulae)

Successful resuscitation of a patient with ECLS requires placement of large cannulae. The most common location for placing these is in the right femoral artery and vein. The venous sheath is long and typically 20-French (7 mm) in diameter. It enters the right femoral vein and extends to the right atrial-inferior vena cava junction. If x-ray is available with fluoroscopy this can be verified. Otherwise this cannula is placed empirically. Because holes are present throughout the length of the distal half of this cannula, adequate venous flow is still possible despite variations in position.

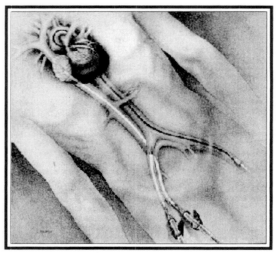

Figure 11-36. *ECLS Catheter.* Illustration compliments of Bard Cardiopulmonary Products, Haverhill, MA.

The arterial cannula is relatively short, ending just below the aortic bifurcation. It may vary in diameter between 16–20-French (5.3-7 mm) depending on the size of the patient. Because limb ischemia is a common complication, select a cannula taking into consideration the patient's likely artery diameter based on his or her body size.[45]

Once support is no longer needed, femoral vein and artery cannulae can be removed in the operating room by a vascular surgeon. Although cannulae can be extracted with percutaneous removal and use of external compression, this is more likely to result in complications.

Percutaneous Extracorporeal Life Support (ECLS)

Percutaneous ECLS is a portable extracorporeal life support machine designed to oxygenate and pump the systemic circulation under urgent conditions via large arterial and venous catheters.

ECLS Recommendations

Emergent institution of ECLS can be considered in rapid circulatory collapse refractory to advanced cardiac life support (ACLS).[31] Symptoms of refractory clinical cardiogenic shock despite inotropes and IABP support also imply the potential need for ECLS if reversible pathology is present or the patient is a candidate for cardiac transplantation. ECLS is most effectively placed in a cardiac catheterization laboratory where cannula position can be verified by x-ray fluoroscopy; it can also be placed without x-ray guidance.

Use of an ECLS system in 81 patients with cardiovascular collapse at our hospital led to a 43.2% survival after 24 hours and 24.7% long-term (>30 day) survival. Patients who had a subsequent surgical or percutaneous treatment were more likely to survive.[46] In 10 patients presenting to the emergency room with the diagnosis of acute myocardial infarction requiring intubation for respiratory failure and CPR for cardiovascular collapse, initiation of ECLS allowed revascularization and long-term survival in four.[47]

CONTRAINDICATIONS AND COMPLICATIONS

In patients without correctable pathology, ECLS initiation can resuscitate the patient neurologically but still lead to a need for subsequent termination of support and death. Thus, consideration of whether a patient may be a potential candidate for cardiac transplant may be appropriate prior to placement of ECLS. Severe aortic regurgitation is also a relative contraindication to ECLS use as reflux into the left ventricle during ECLS support could aggravate pulmonary edema and increase myocardial oxygen consumption.

Even more than with IABP placement, peripheral vascular disease may prevent percutaneous insertion of the large cannulae required. Complications include vascular hemorrhage, leg ischemia, or aortic dissection.[48]

CONTRAINDICATIONS TO ECLS

- No correctable pathology
- Unwitnessed arrest, prolonged CPR
- Severe aortic regurgitation
- Obstructive peripheral vascular disease with inability to insert cannulas

---

Technique for ECLS Insertion

1. Percutaneous access into femoral artery and femoral or internal jugular vein.

2. Dilate femoral artery with either successive dilators (8-French, 14-French, or 16-20-French cannula) or direct exchange for arterial cannula. Have assistant apply gentle back-and-forth motion of guide wire to detect kinking of wire during cannula placement.

3. Insert 0.038 inch stiff J-type wire into vein and dilate with venous 14-French dilator. Insert venous cannula to estimate of mid-right atrium.

4. Give heparin. Eliminate all air in arterial cannula by circulating saline through arteriovenous crossbridge with arterial tubing clamp open. Aspirate remaining air through distal arterial tubing stopcock.

5. Connect cannulas to system and initiate pumping as per perfusion protocol. Sew cannulas into place with thick suture material.

Location	Venous Cannulation	Arterial Cannulation	Rationale
Cath Lab	Femoral	Femoral	Sheaths in place; Fluoroscopy readily available
SICU after CABG	Jugular/RA	Femoral/ Asc. Ao.	Open chest is suspected; tamponade
ER	Jugular	Femoral	No fluoroscopy Possible volume loss situation
ICU/CCU	Jugular/ Femoral	Femoral	No fluoroscopy ? CVP line in jugular ? Post PTCA sheaths in place
Floor	Jugular	Femoral	No fluoroscopy

The anatomic site of venous and arterial cannulation can depend on the facilities immediately available at the time of cardiac decompensation or arrest.

Left Ventricular Assist Device (LVAD)

An LVAD unloads and assumes the pumping function of the left ventricle to maintain adequate systemic blood flow with little or no ventricular contribution. The device may support the left (LVAD) and/or the right (RVAD) ventricle and can deliver total output of up to 10 L/min. VAD insertion, however, requires a sternotomy, advanced personnel training, equipment monitoring, and availability of the device. Recent long-term support with implantable LVAD's suggest that chronic support as an alternative to heart transplantation may be possible in the future with these devices.[49, 50]

In patients implanted with the LVAD, exercise rehabilitation may improve the overall physical state of the patient to improve their transplant operative survival and long-term prognosis.

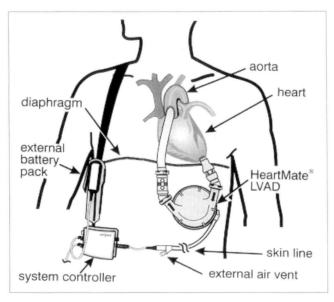

Figure 11-37. *Vented electric LVAD.* Illustration complements of Thermo Cardiosystems Incorporated, Woburn, MA.

aorta

heart

diaphragm

external battery pack

HeartMate® LVAD

skin line

system controller

external air vent

The above diagram indicates the typical placement of a vented electric LVAD.[51] For simplicity, only one battery under the right axilla is shown although an additional battery under the left axilla is also used. Batteries typically last eight hours before requiring replacement and recharging. The LVAD itself is in a pre-peritoneal pocket by the rectus sheath. The only penetration of the skin barrier is by the exit of the power wires and vent tube typically in the right or left lower quadrant. At rest, the LVAD acts as a series pump with nearly all flow from the left ventricle entering the LVAD prior to ejection into the patient's ascending aorta. With exercise, increased loading and contractility of the left ventricle lead to parallel flow out of the native aortic valve that may contribute to flow ejected by the LVAD.[49]

Future Directions

Improvements in heart failure therapy are currently under intense clinical investigation. Greater use of evidence based approaches to favorably affect left ventricular disease progression should reduce morbidity and mortality. Multidisciplinary strategies that encourage patients to be active participants in their care may reduce the occurrence of decompensated heart failure and possibly improve survival.

It is likely that progression of left ventricular dysfunction will be treated with new classes of medications. These could include drugs that block vasopressin or endothelin effects or those which promote nitric oxide production. Angiotensin II receptor blockers may have an added role to ACE inhibition.

Prevention of sudden death will include use of automatic implantable cardioversion defibrillators. These devices will become smaller and the cost of implantation will become less. Ultimately, many patients with chronic heart failure will still develop end-stage left ventricular pump dysfunction and benefit from heart replacement therapy. Although the gold standard at this time is cardiac transplantation, in the future, options may include permanent left ventricular assist device placement, xeno-transplant with hearts from genetically engineered animals, or finally gene therapy tailored to return the structure of a failing heart to normal.[52, 53]

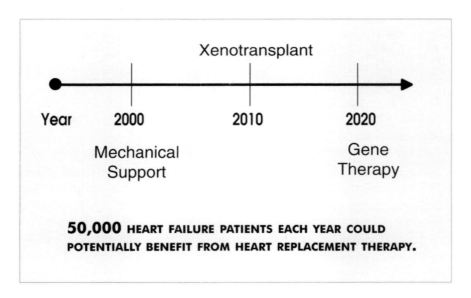

Year   2000   2010   2020

Xenotransplant

Mechanical   Gene
Support   Therapy

50,000 HEART FAILURE PATIENTS EACH YEAR COULD
POTENTIALLY BENEFIT FROM HEART REPLACEMENT THERAPY.

Chapter 11 Case Scenarios

SCENARIO #1

MEDICAL HISTORY

22-year-old female with two-week history of rapidly progressive shortness of breath, weakness and fatigue. Normal vaginal delivery of first pregnancy three months prior. No significant history of alcohol use.

PHYSICAL EXAM

BP: 100/80
HR: 120, regular
T: Afebrile
JVP: 15 cm H_2O
CHEST: Ronchi, no rales, wheezes
COR: Summation gallop; no murmur
EXT: Trace edema bilaterally
CXR: Mild cardiomegaly,
     mild pulmonary congestion

Urine Toxicology Screen: negative
Echo: severe global hypokinesis
     (ED dim=6.0)

MEDICATIONS

Transferred on dobutamine (4µg/kg/min), digoxin, furosemide with persistent dyspnea and only moderate diuresis.

Question 1a

What would you recommend for this patient?

a) Right heart catheterization

b) Left heart catheterization

c) Radionuclide wall motion

d) Endomyocardial biopsy

e) Thallium stress test

Scenario #1 Continued

Therapy

The patient underwent a right heart catheterization and her initial hemodynamics were calculated.

Initial Hemodynamics

BP = 100/80
HR = 110
RA = 16
PA = 45/28
PCW = 25
Cardiac Index = 1.6 L/min/m^2

Question 1b

Evaluate the therapies listed below for this inpatient:

a. Very helpful
b. Marginally helpful
c. Not helpful or potentially harmful

_____ 1. nitroprusside

_____ 2. nitroglycerin SL

_____ 3. nitroglycerin IV

_____ 4. nitroglycerin topical

_____ 5. dopamine

_____ 6. amlodipine

_____ 7. β-blocker

_____ 8. milrinone

_____ 9. ACE Inhibitor

_____ 10. amiodarone

Scenario #2

Medical History and Physical Exam

A 51-year-old male experienced an abrupt onset of shortness of breath. Paramedics witnessed an episode of ventricular fibrillation, defibrillated the patient, and transported him. ECG showed sinus tachycardia at a rate of 115 bpm and an extensive acute anterior myocardial infarction with up to 10 mm of precordial S T elevation. The patient required defibrillation and intubation for a second episode of ventricular fibrillation while in the emergency room. Progressive hypotension developed despite being given dopamine at 20 µg/kg/min with a systolic blood pressure of 70 mm Hg.

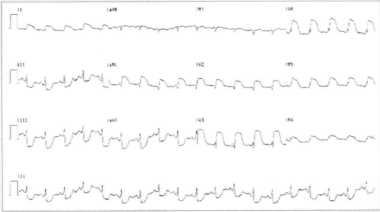

Figure 11-38. *Scenario #2a ECG.*

Question 2a

How would you proceed?

a) IV thrombolysis

b) Echocardiogram

c) IABP and cardiac catheterization

d) IV epinephrine

e) IV milrinone

f) IV nitroglycerin

SCENARIO #2 CONTINUED

THERAPY

The patient was emergently transferred to the cardiac catheter-ization laboratory. Intra-aortic balloon pumping (IABP) through the left femoral artery was initiated. Coro-nary angiography from the right femoral artery re-vealed a totally occluded left main

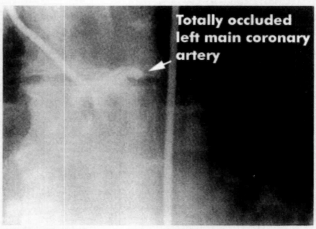

Totally occluded left main coronary artery

Figure 11-39. *Scenario #2b catheterization showing a totally occluded left main coronary artery.*

coronary artery and a 50% right coronary artery stenosis. No collaterals to the left coronary artery were noted by angiography.

Consultation with cardiac surgery after diagnostic angiography noted both an unacceptably high cardiovascular risk associated with urgent bypass surgery and an uncertain patient neurologic status. The left main was initially dilated with a 3.0 mm balloon approximately two hours after the onset of symptoms. Despite IABP placement and inotropic support, the mean blood pressure remained at 50 mm Hg.

Question 2b

What would you do now?

a) Repeat percutaneous revascularization

b) IV epinephrine

c) Placement of percutaneous extracorporeal life support (ECLS)

d) Left ventricular assist device

SCENARIO #2 CONTINUED

The patient was placed on ECLS with exchange of the IABP for the ECLS arterial cannula over a wire, and the venous cannula was inserted from the left femoral vein. Dopamine was immediately discontinued with maintenance of a mean arterial pressure of 90 mm Hg and a ECLS flow rate of 4 L/min. Repeat angiography revealed severely stenosed proximal circumflex and left anterior descending (LAD) arteries. Dilation was repeated on the left main, proximal circumflex, and the left anterior descending

arteries. Following this, the left main and LAD were seen to be patent. The left circumflex, however, demonstrated threatened closure despite repeated inflations requiring stent placement. Despite revascularization, the patient remained ECLS-dependent.

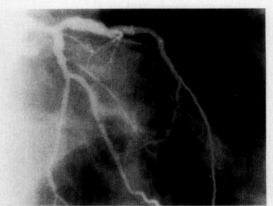

Figure 11-40. *Scenario #2c, repeat angiography reveals patent left main, proximal circumflex, and left anterior descending arteries.*

Question 2c

What would you do now?

a) Continue ECLS support

b) Emergent bypass surgery

c) Left ventricular assist device (bridge to transplant)

d) Withdraw support

See Appendix for solutions.

References

Part I - The Problem of Heart Failure

INTRODUCTION

1. Katz AM. Molecular biology in cardiology, a paradigmatic shift. J.Mol.Cell Cardiol.1988; 20:355-366.

CHAPTER 1 — POPULATION

1. American Heart Association. Heart and Stroke Facts.1998.
2. Gillum RF. Epidemiology of heart failure in the United States. Am.Heart J. 1993; 126:1042-1047.
3. Ho KK, Pinsky JL, Kannel WB, Levy D. The epidemiology of heart failure: the Framingham Study. J.Am.Coll.Cardiol. 1993; 22:6A-13A.
4. McKee PA, Castelli WP, McNamara PM, Kannel WB. The natural history of congestive heart failure: the Framingham study. N.Engl.J.Med. 1971; 285:1441-1446.
5. Senni M, Tribouilloy CM, Rodeheffer RJ, Jacobsen SJ, Evans JM, Bailey KR, Redfield MM. Congestive heart failure in the community: trends in incidence and survival in a 10-year period. Arch.Intern.Med. 1999; 159:29-34.
6. Centers for Disease Control. Mortality from congestive heart failure in the United States, 1980-1990. Morbidity and Mortality Weekly Report 1994; 5:77-81.
7. National Heart Lung and Blood Institute. Congestive Heart Failure in the United States: A New Epidemic. 1993.
8. Gheorghiade M, Bonow RO. Chronic heart failure in the United States: a manifestation of coronary artery disease. Circulation. 1998; 97: 282-289.
9. Ho KK, Anderson KM, Kannel WB, Grossman W, Levy D. Survival after the onset of congestive heart failure in Framingham Heart Study subjects. Circulation. 1993; 88:107-115.
10. The sixth report of the Joint National Committee on prevention, detection, evaluation, and treatment of high blood pressure. Arch.Intern.Med. 1997; 157:2413-2446.
11. Uretsky BF, Sheahan RG. Primary prevention of sudden cardiac death in heart failure: will the solution be shocking? J.Am.Coll.Cardiol. 1997; 30:1589-1597.
12. Massie BM, Shah NB. Evolving trends in the epidemiologic factors of heart failure: rationale for preventive strategies and comprehensive disease management. Am.Heart J. 1997; 133:703-712.
13. Luu M, Stevenson WG, Stevenson LW, Baron K, Walden J. Diverse mechanisms of unexpected cardiac arrest in advanced heart failure. Circulation. 1989; 80:1675-1680.
14. Vasan RS, Larson MG, Benjamin EJ, Evans JC, Reiss CK, Levy D. Congestive heart failure in subjects with normal versus reduced left ventricular ejection fraction: prevalence and mortality in a population- based cohort. J. Am.Coll.Cardiol. 1999; 33:1948-1955.
15. Adams KFJ, Sueta CA, Gheorghiade M, O'Connor CM, Schwartz TA, Koch GG, Uretsky B, Swedberg K, McKenna W, Soler-Soler J, Califf RM. Gender differences in survival in advanced heart failure. Insights from the FIRST study. Circulation. 1999; 99:1816-1821.
16. Scognamiglio R, Avogaro A, Casara D, Crepaldi C, Marin M, Palisi M, Mingardi R, Erle G, Fasoli G, Dalla VS. Myocardial dysfunction and adrenergic cardiac innervation in patients with insulin-dependent diabetes mellitus. J.Am.Coll.Cardiol. 1998; 31:404-412.
17. O'Connell JB, Bristow MR. Economic impact of heart failure in the United States: time for a different approach. J.Heart Lung Transplant. 1994; 13:S107-S112.
18. Hurst JW. Paul Dudley White: to know him better. Am.J.Cardiol. 1985; 56:169-177.

CHAPTER 2 — INDIVIDUAL

1. Levine SA. Clinical heart disease. Nature and treatment of congestive heart failure. 4th ed. Philadelphia: WB Saunders, 1951; 291.
2. McKee PA, Castelli WP, McNamara PM, Kannel WB. The natural history of congestive heart failure: the Framingham study. N.Engl.J.Med. 1971; 285:1441-1446.
3. Stevenson LW, Perloff JK. The limited reliability of physical signs for estimating hemodynamics in chronic heart failure. JAMA 1989; 261:884-888.
4. Butman SM, Ewy GA, Standen JR, Kern KB, Hahn E. Bedside cardiovascular examination in patients with severe chronic heart failure: importance of rest or inducible jugular venous distension. J.Am.Coll.Cardiol. 1993; 22:968-974.

CHAPTER 3 — CIRCULATION

1. Grossman W. Cardiac catheterization and angiography. 5 ed. Baltimore: Williams and Wilkins, 1996; 281-295.
2. Somlyo AP, Somlyo AV. Smooth muscle structure and function. In: Fozzard HA, Haber E, Jennings RB, Katz AM, Morgan HE, editors. The heart and cardiovascular system. 2 ed. New York: Raven, 1992; 1295-1324.
3. Peterson KL, Skloven D, Ludbrook P, Uther JB, Ross JJ. Comparison of isovolumic and ejection phase indices of myocardial performance in man. Circulation. 1974; 49:1088-1101.
4. Ross JJ. Applications and limitations of end-systolic measures of ventricular performance. Fed.Proc. 1984; 43:2418-2422.
5. Wroblewski H, Norgaard T, Haunso S, Kastrup J. Microvascular distensibility in two different vascular beds in idiopathic dilated cardiomyopathy. Am.J.Physiol. 1995; 269:H1973-H1980.
6. Jaski BE, Fifer MA, Wright RF, Braunwald E, Colucci WS. Positive inotropic and vasodilator actions of milrinone in patients with severe congestive heart failure. Dose-response relationships and comparison to nitroprusside. J.Clin.Invest. 1985; 75:643-649.
7. Cohn JN, Levine TB, Olivari MT, Garberg V, Lura D, Francis GS, et al. Plasma norepinephrine as a guide to prognosis in patients with chronic congestive heart failure. N.Engl.J.Med. 1984; 311:819-823.
8. Cohn JN, Levine TB, Francis GS, Goldsmith S. Neurohumoral control mechanisms in congestive heart failure. Am.Heart J. 1981; 102:509-514.
9. Daly PA, Sole MJ. Myocardial catecholamines and the pathophysiology of heart failure. Circulation. 1990; 82:I35-I43.
10. Colucci WS, Denniss AR, Leatherman GF, Quigg RJ, Ludmer PL, Marsh JD, et al. Intracoronary infusion of dobutamine to patients with and without severe congestive heart failure. Dose-response relationships, correlation with circulating catecholamines, and effect of phosphodiesterase inhibition. J.Clin.Invest. 1988; 81:1103-1110.
11. Levine TB, Francis GS, Goldsmith SR, Cohn JN. The neurohumoral and hemodynamic response to orthostatic tilt in patients with congestive heart failure. Circulation. 1983; 67:1070-1075.
12. Ferguson DW, Abboud FM, Mark AL. Selective impairment of baroreflex-mediated vasoconstrictor responses in patients with ventricular dysfunction. Circulation. 1984; 69:451-460.
13. Imperato-McGinley J, Gautier T, Ehlers K, Zullo MA, Goldstein DS, Vaughan EDJ. Reversibility of catecholamine-induced dilated cardiomyopathy in a child with a pheochromocytoma. N.Engl.J.Med. 1987; 316:793-797.
14. Dzau VJ, Colucci WS, Hollenberg NK, Williams GH. Relation of the renin-angiotensin-aldosterone system to clinical state in congestive heart failure. Circulation. 1981; 63:645-651.
15. Hirsch AT, Pinto YM, Schunkert H, Dzau VJ. Potential role of the tissue renin-angiotensin system in the pathophysiology of congestive heart failure. Am.J.Cardiol. 1990; 66:22D-30D.

16. Delcayre C, Silvestre J. Aldosterone and the heart: towards a physiological function? Cardiovasc.Res. 1999; 43:7-12.

17. MacFadyen RJ, Barr CS, Struthers AD. Aldosterone blockade reduces vascular collagen turnover, improves heart rate variability and reduces early morning rise in heart rate in heart failure patients. Cardiovasc.Res. 1997; 35:30-34.

18. Wang W, McClain JM, Zucker IH. Aldosterone reduces baroreceptor discharge in the dog. Hypertension. 1992; 19:270-277.

19. Swedberg K, Eneroth P, Kjekshus J, Wilhelmsen L. Hormones regulating cardiovascular function in patients with severe congestive heart failure and their relation to mortality. CONSENSUS Trial Study Group. Circulation. 1990; 82:1730-1736.

20. Pitt B, Zannad F, Remme WJ, Cody R, Castaigne A, Perez A, Palensky J, Wittes J. The effect of spironolactone on morbidity and mortality in patients with severe heart failure. N.Engl.J.Med. 1999; 341:709-717.

21. Dzau VJ. Tissue renin-angiotensin system: physiologic and pharmacologic implications. Introduction. Circulation. 1988; 77:I1-I3.

22. Zimmerman BG, Sybertz EJ, Wong PC. Interaction between sympathetic and renin-angiotensin system. J.Hypertens. 1984; 2:581-587.

23. Riegger GA, Kochsiek K. Vasopressin, renin and norepinephrine levels before and after captopril administration in patients with congestive heart failure due to idiopathic dilated cardiomyopathy. Am.J.Cardiol. 1986; 58:300-303.

24. Zisman LS. Inhibiting tissue angiotensin-converting enzyme: a pound of flesh without the blood? Circulation. 1998; 98:2788-2790.

25. Packer M. The neurohormonal hypothesis: a theory to explain the mechanism of disease progression in heart failure. J.Am.Coll.Cardiol. 1992; 20:248-254.

26. Packer M, Carver JR, Rodeheffer RJ, Ivanhoe RJ, DiBianco R, Zeldis SM, et al. Effect of oral milrinone on mortality in severe chronic heart failure. The PROMISE Study Research Group. N.Engl.J.Med. 1991; 325:1468-1475.

27. Dies F, Krell M.J., Whitlow P, Liang C, Goldenberg I, Applefeld M, et al. Intermittent dobutamine in ambulatory outpatients with chronic cardiac failure. Circulation. 1998; Abstract.

28. Packer M, Rouleau JL, Swedberg K, Pitt B, Fisher L, Klepper M. Effect of Flosequinan on survival in chronic heart failure: preliminary results of the PROFILE study. Circulation. 1993; 88 (Supp I):I-301 Abstract.

29. Katz AM. Heart Failure. In: Fozzard HA, Haber E, Jennings RB, Katz AM, Morgan HE, editors. The heart and cardiovascular system. 2 ed. New York: Raven, 1992; 333-353.

30. Fazio S, Sabatini D, Capaldo B, Vigorito C, Giordano A, Guida R, et al. A preliminary study of growth hormone in the treatment of dilated cardiomyopathy. N.Engl.J.Med. 1996; 334:809-814.

31. Cohn JN. Vasodilators in heart failure. Conclusions from V-HeFT II and rationale for V-HeFT III. Drugs 1994; 47 (Suppl 4):47-57; discussion 57-8:47-57.

32. Francis GS, Benedict C, Johnstone DE, Kirlin PC, Nicklas J, Liang CS, et al. Comparison of neuroendocrine activation in patients with left ventricular dysfunction with and without congestive heart failure. A substudy of the Studies of Left Ventricular Dysfunction (SOLVD). Circulation. 1990; 82:1724-1729.

33. Tsuchimochi H, Kurimoto F, Leki K, Koyama H, Takaku F, Kawana M, Kimata S, Yazaki Y. Atrial natriuretic peptide distribution in fetal and failed adult human hearts. Circulation. 1988; 78:920-927.

34. McMullen ET. Anatomy of a physiological discovery: William Harvey and the circulation of the blood. J.R.Soc.Med. 1995; 88:491-498.

CHAPTER 4 — ORGAN

1. Hoffman EA, Ritman EL. Invariant total heart volume in the intact thorax. Am.J.Physiol. 1985; 249:H883-H890.
2. Senni M, Redfield MM. Congestive heart failure in elderly patients. Mayo Clin.Proc. 1997; 72:453-460.
3. Bier AJ, Eichacker PQ, Sinoway LI, Terribile SM, Strom JA, Keefe DL. Acute cardiogenic pulmonary edema: clinical and noninvasive evaluation. Angiology. 1988; 39:211-218.
4. Mirsky I. Left ventricular stresses in the intact human heart. Biophysic. Journal. 1969; 9:189-208.
5. Jaski BE, Serruys PW. Epicardial wall motion and left ventricular function during coronary graft angioplasty in humans. J.Am.Coll.Cardiol. 1985; 6:695-700.
6. Colucci WS, Braunwald E. Pathophysiology of heart failure. In: Braunwald E, editor. Heart disease: a textbook of cardiovascular medicine. 5 ed. Philadelphia: WB Saunders, 1997; 394-420.
7. Grossman W, Jones D, McLaurin LP. Wall stress and patterns of hypertrophy in the human left ventricle. J.Clin.Invest. 1975; 56:56-64.
8. Gorlin R. Treatment of congestive heart failure: where are we going? Circulation. 1987; 75:IV108-IV111.
9. Pouleur H. Abnormalities in cardiac relaxation and other forms of diastolic dysfunction. In: Hosenpud JD, Greenberg B, eds. Congestive heart failure: pathophysiology, diagnosis and comprehensive approach to management. New York: Springer-Verlag, 1993: 68.
10. Brutsaert DL, Rademakers FE, Sys SU. Triple control of relaxation: implications in cardiac disease. Circulation. 1984; 69:190-196.
11. Auricchio A, Stellbrink C, Sack S, Block M, Vogt J, Bakker P, Mortensen P, Klein H. The Pacing Therapies for Congestive Heart Failure (PATH-CHF) study: rationale, design, and endpoints of a prospective randomized multicenter study. Am. J. Cardiol. 1999; 83:130D-135D.

CHAPTER 5 — CELL

1. Streeter DDJ, Spotnitz HM, Patel DP, Ross JJ, Sonnenblick EH. Fiber orientation in the canine left ventricle during diastole and systole. 1924; 1-47.
2. Beltrami CA, Finato N, Rocco M, Feruglio GA, C. Puricelli C, Cigola E, Quaini F, Sonnenblick EH, Olivetti G, Anversa P. Structural basis of end-stage failure in ischemic cardiomyopathy in humans. Circulation. 1994; 89:151-163.
3. Roberts WC, Siegel RJ, McManus BM. Idiopathic dilated cardiomyopathy: analysis of 152 necropsy patients. Am.J.Cardiol. 1987; 60: 1340-1355.
4. Katz AM. Molecular and cellular basis of contraction. In: Braunwald E, Colucci WS, editors. Atlas of heart diseases. Heart failure: cardiac function and dysfunction. Philadelphia: Mosby, 1995.
5. Braunwald E, Ross J, Sonnenblick E. Mechanisms of contraction of the normal and failing heart. Boston: Little, Brown and Company, 1976; 3.
6. Schauf, Charles. Human Physiology, Foundations and Frontiers. St. Louis: Times Mirror/ Mosby College Publishing, 1990; 293.
7. Opie LH. Mechanisms of cardiac contraction and relaxation. In:Braunwald E, editor. Heart disease: a textbook of cardiovascular medicine. 5 ed. Philadelphia: WB Saunders, 1997; 360-393.
8. Briman NA, Levine HJ. Contractile element work: a major determinant of myocardial oxygen consumption. J.Clin.Invest. 1964; 43:1397-1408.
9. Tanser PH. Hypertrophy to failure. J. Hum. Hypertens. 1994; 8 (Suppl 1): S17-S20.
10. Wangler RD, Peters KG, Marcus ML, Tomanek RJ. Effects of duration and severity of arterial hypertension and cardiac hypertrophy on coronary vasodilator reserve. Circ.Res. 1982; 51:10-18.

11. Gorcsan J, Feldman AM, Kormos RL, Mandarino WA, Demetris AJ and Batista RJ. Heterogeneous immediate effects of partial left ventriculectomy on cardiac performance. Circulation. 1998; 97:839-842.

12. Morgan JP, Chesebro JH, Pluth JR, Puga FJ, Schaff HV. Intracellular calcium transients in human working myocardium as detected with aequorin. J.Am.Coll.Cardiol. 1984; 3:410-418.

13. Gilbert EM, Abraham WT, Olsen S, Hattler B, White M, Mealy P, et al. Comparative hemodynamic, left ventricular functional, and antiadrenergic effects of chronic treatment with metoprolol versus carvedilol in the failing heart. Circulation. 1996; 94:2817-2825.

14. Bristow MR, Ginsburg R, Minobe W, Cubicciotti RS, Sageman WS, Lurie K, Billingham ME, Harrison DC, Stinson EB. Decreased catecholamine sensitivity and beta-adrenergic-receptor density in failing human hearts. N.Engl.J.Med. 1982; 307:205-211 .

15. Berne RM, Levy MN. Cardiovascular physiology. St. Louis: Mosby, 1997:171-179.

16. Somlyo AP, Somlyo AV. Smooth muscle structure and function. In: Fozzard HA, Haber E, Jennings RB, Katz AM, Morgan HE, editors. The heart and cardiovascular system. 2 ed. New York: Raven, 1992;1295-1324.

17. Morgan JP, Morgan KG. Calcium and cardiovascular function. Intracellular calcium levels during contraction and relaxation of mammalian cardiac and vascular smooth muscle as detected with aequorin. Am.J.Med. 1984; 77:33-46.

18. Katz AM. Regulation of myocardial contractility 1958-1983: an odyssey. J.Am.Coll.Cardiol. 1983; 1:42-51.

19. Shabb JB, Corbin JD. Protein phosphorylation. In: Fozzard HA, Haber E, Jennings RB, Katz AM, Morgan HE, editors. The heart and cardiovascular system: Scientific foundations. 2 ed. New York: Raven, 1992;1505-1524.

CHAPTER 6 — SARCOMERE

1. Katz AM. Molecular and cellular basis of contraction. In: Braunwald E, Colucci WS, editors. Atlas of heart diseases. Heart failure: cardiac function and dysfunction. Philadelphia: Mosby and Current Medicine, 1995: 1.0-2.0.

2. Ganong WF. Excitable tissue: muscle. In: Review of medical physiology. 17 ed. Norwalk: Appleton & Lange, 1995;56-74.

3. Katz AM. Physiology of the heart. New York: Raven Press, 1992; 153-180.

4. Bowman P, Haikala H, Paul RJ. Levosimendan, a calcium sensitizer in cardiac muscle, induces relaxation in coronary smooth muscle through calcium desensitization. J Pharmacol.Exp.Ther. 1999; 288:316-325.

CHPATER 7 — GENE

1. Glennon PE, Sugden PH, Poole-Wilson PA. Cellular mechanisms of cardiac hypertrophy. Br.Heart J. 1995; 73:496-499.

2. Lee TH, Hamilton MA, Stevenson LW, Moriguchi JD, Fonarow GC, Child JS, et al. Impact of left ventricular cavity size on survival in advanced heart failure. Am.J.Cardiol. 1993; 72:672-676.

3. Beltrami CA, Finato N, Rocco M, Feruglio GA, Puricelli C, Cigola E, Quaini F, Sonnenblick EH, Olivetti G, Anversa P. Structural basis of end-stage failure in ischemic cardiomyopathy in humans. Circulation. 1994; 89:151-163.

4. Roberts WC, Siegel RJ and McManus BM. Idiopathic dilated cardiomyopathy: analysis of 152 necropsy patients. Am.J.Cardiol. 1987; 60:1340-1355.

5. Olivetti G, Abbi R, Quaini F, Kajstura J, Cheng W, Nitahara JA, et al. Apoptosis in the failing human heart. N.Engl.J.Med. 1997; 336:1131-1141.

6. Blum A, Miller H. Role of cytokines in heart failure. Am.Heart J. 1998; 135:181-186.

7. McKenna CJ, Sugrue DD, Kwon HM, Sangiorgi G, Carlson PJ, Mahon N, McCann HA, Edwards WD, Holmes DRJ, Schwartz RS. Histopathologic changes in asymptomatic relatives of patients with idiopathic dilated cardiomyopathy. Am.J. Cardiol. 1999; 83:281-283, A6.

8. Sharov VG, Sabbah HN, Shimoyama H, Goussev AV, Lesch M, Goldstein S. Evidence of cardiocyte apoptosis in myocardium of dogs with chronic heart failure. Am.J.Pathol. 1996; 148:141-149.

9. Boluyt MO, Bing OH, Lakatta EG. The ageing spontaneously hypertensive rat as a model of the transition from stable compensated hypertrophy to heart failure. Eur.Heart J. 1995; 16 (Suppl N):19-30.

10. Francis GS. TNF-alpha and heart failure : the difference between proof of principle and hypothesis testing. Circulation. 1999; 99:3213-3214.

11. Bristow MR. Tumor necrosis factor-alpha and cardiomyopathy. Circulation. 1998; 97:1340-1341.

12. Satoh M, Nakamura M, Tamura G, Makita S, Segawa I, Tashiro A, et al. Inducible nitric oxide synthase and tumor necrosis factor-alpha in myocardium in human dilated cardiomyopathy. J.Am.Coll.Cardiol. 1997; 29:716-724.

13. Deswal A, Bozkurt B, Seta Y, Parilti-Eiswirth S, Hayes FA, Blosch C, Mann DL. Safety and efficacy of a soluble P75 tumor necrosis factor receptor (Enbrel, etanercept) in patients with advanced heart failure. Circulation. 1999; 99:3224-3226.

CHAPTER 8 — MOLECULE

1. Niimura H, Bachinski LL, Sangwatanaroj S, Watkins H, Chudley AE, McKenna W, Kristinsson A, Roberts R, Sole M, MaronBJ, Seidman JG, Seidman CE. Mutations in the gene for cardiac myosin-binding protein C and late- onset familial hypertrophic cardiomyopathy. N.Engl.J.Med. 1998; 338:1248-1257.

2. Spirito P, Seidman CE, McKenna WJ, Maron BJ. The management of hypertrophic cardiomyopathy. N.Engl.J.Med. 1997; 336:775-785.

3. Epstein ND, Cohn GM, Cyran F, Fananapazir L. Differences in clinical expression of hypertrophic cardiomyopathy associated with two distinct mutations in the beta-myosin heavy chain gene. A 908Leu----Val mutation and a 403Arg----Gln mutation. Circulation. 1992; 86:345-352.

4. Katz AM. Regulation of myocardial contractility 1958-1983: an odyssey. J.Am.Coll.Cardiol. 1983; 1:42-51.

5. Hasenfuss G, Meyer M, Schillinger W, Preuss M, Pieske B, Just H. Calcium handling proteins in the failing human heart. Basic Res.Cardiol. 1997; 92 (Suppl 1):87-93.

Part II - The Management of Heart Failure

CHAPTER 9 — DIAGNOSIS

1. Konstam MA, Dracup K, Baker DW. Heart failure: Evaluation and care of patients with left-ventricular systolic dysfunction. US Department of Health and Human Services 1994; 11.

2. Richardson P, McKenna W, Bristow M, Maisch B, Mautner B, O'Connell J, Olsen E, Thiene G, Goodwin J, Gyarfas I, Martin I, Nordet P. Report of the 1995 world health organization/international society and federation of cardiology task force on the definition and classification of cardiomyopathies. Circulation. 1996; 93:841-842.

3. Kloner RA, Bolli R, Marban E, Reinlib L, Braunwald E., and Participants. Medical and cellular implications of stunning, hibernation, and preconditioning. An NHLBI workshop. Circulation. 1998; 97:1848-1867.

4. Wijns W, Vatner SF, Camici PG. Hibernating myocardium. N.Engl.J Med. 1998; 339:173-181.

5. Senior R, Kaul S, Lahiri A. Myocardial viability on echocardiography predicts long-term survival after revascularization in patients with ischemic congestive heart failure. J. Am.Coll.Cardiol. 1999; 33:1848-1854.

6. Cornel JH, Bax JJ, Elhendy A, Maat AP, Kimman GJ, Geleijnse ML, Rambaldi R, Boersma E, Fioretti PM. Biphasic response to dobutamine predicts improvement of global left ventricular function after surgical revascularization in patients with stable coronary artery disease: implications of time course of recovery on diagnostic accuracy. J.Am.Coll.Cardiol. 1998; 31:1002-1010.

7. Afridi I, Qureshi U, Kopelen HA, Winters WL, Zoghbi WA. Serial changes in response of hibernating myocardium to inotropic stimulation after revascularization: a dobutamine echocardiographic study. J.Am.Coll.Cardiol. 1997; 30:1233-1240.

8. Geleijnse ML, Salustri A, Marwick TH, Fioretti PM. Should the diagnosis of coronary artery disease be based on the evaluation of myocardial function or perfusion? Eur.Heart J. 1997; 18 (Suppl D):D68-77.

9. Brown KA. Do stress echocardiography and myocardial perfusion imaging have the same ability to identify the low-risk patient with known or suspected coronary artery disease? Am.J.Cardiol. 1998; 81:1050-1053.

10. Hosenpud JD. The cardiomyopathies. In: Hosenpud JD, Greenberg BH. Congestive heart failure: Pathophysiology, diagnosis, and comprehensive approach to mangement. New York: Springer-Verlag, 1994;196-222.

11. Grunig E, Tasman JA, Kucherer H, Franz W, Kubler W and Katus HA. Frequency and phenotypes of familial dilated cardiomyopathy. J.Am.Coll.Cardiol. 1998; 31:186-194.

12. Maeda M, Holder E, Lowes B, Valent S, Bies RD. Dilated cardiomyopathy associated with deficiency of the cytoskeletal protein metavinculin. Circulation. 1997; 95:17-20.

13. Muntoni F, Cau M, Ganau A, Congiu R, Arvedi G, Mateddu A, et al. Brief report: deletion of the dystrophin muscle-promoter region associated with X-linked dilated cardiomyopathy. N.Engl.J.Med. 1993; 329:921-925.

14. Fadic R, Sunada Y, Waclawik AJ, Buck S, Lewandoski PJ, Campbell KP, et al. Brief report: deficiency of a dystrophin-associated glycoprotein (adhalin) in a patient with muscular dystrophy and cardiomyopathy. N.Engl.J.Med. 1996; 334:362-366.

15. Powell LW, Isselbacher KJ. Hemochromatosis. In: Fauci AS, Braunwald E, Isselbacher KJ. Harrison's principles of internal medicine. New York: McGraw-Hill, 1998; 2149-2152.

16. Bothwell TH, MacPhail AP. Hereditary hemochromatosis: etiologic, pathologic, and clinical aspects. Semin.Hematol. 1998; 35:55-71.

17. Mason JW, O'Connell JB, Herskowitz A, Rose NR, McManus BM, Billingham ME, et al. A clinical trial of immunosuppressive therapy for myocarditis. The Myocarditis Treatment Trial Investigators. N.Engl.J.Med. 1995; 333:269-275.

18. Dembitsky WP, Moore CH, Holman WL, Jaski BE, Moreno-Cabral RJ, Adamson RM, Daily PO, Moreno-Cabral CE. Successful mechanical circulatory support for noncoronary shock. J.Heart Lung Transplant. 1992; 11:129-135.

19. Witlin AG, Mabie WC, Sibai BM. Peripartum cardiomyopathy: an ominous diagnosis. Am.J.Obstet.Gynecol. 1997; 176:182-188.

20. Wenger NK, Speroff L, Packard B. Cardiovascular health and disease in women. N. Engl. J. Med.1993; 329:247-256.

21. Rabbani LE, Wang PJ, Couper GL, Friedman PL. Time course of improvement in ventricular function after ablation of incessant automatic atrial tachycardia. Am.Heart J. 1991; 121:816-819.

22. Mason JW, O'Connell JB. Clinical merit of endomyocardial biopsy. Circulation. 1989; 79:971-979.

23. Nishimura RA, Tajik AJ. Evaluation of diastolic filling of left ventricle in health and disease: Doppler echocardiography is the clinician's Rosetta Stone. J.Am.Coll.Cardiol. 1997; 30:8-18.

24. Garcia MJ, Thomas JD, Klein AL. New Doppler echocardiographic applications for the study of diastolic function. J.Am.Coll.Cardiol. 1998; 32:865-875.

25. Maron BJ, Gardin JM, Flack JM, Gidding SS, Kurosaki TT, Bild DE. Prevalence of hypertrophic cardiomyopathy in a general population of young adults. Echocardiographic analysis of 4111 subjects in the CARDIA Study. Coronary Artery Risk Development in (Young) Adults. Circulation. 1995; 92:785-789.

26. Spirito P, Seidman CE, McKenna WJ, Maron BJ. The management of hypertrophic cardiomyopathy. N.Engl.J.Med. 1997; 336:775-785.

27. Kushwaha SS, Fallon JT, Fuster V. Restrictive cardiomyopathy. N.Engl.J.Med. 1997; 336:267-276.

28. Kyle RA, Gertz MA, Greipp PR, Witzig TE, Lust JA, Lacy MQ, Therneau TM. A trial of three regimens for primary amyloidosis: colchicine alone, melphalan and prednisone, and melphalan, prednisone, and colchicine. N.Engl.J.Med. 1997; 336:1202-1207.

29. Pelosi FJ, Capehart J, Roberts WC. Effectiveness of cardiac transplantation for primary (AL) cardiac amyloidosis. Am.J.Cardiol. 1997; 79:532-535.

30. Grossman W. Cardiac catheterization, angiography, and intervention. 5 ed. Philadelphia: Lea & Febiger, 1996; 668-673.

31. Carabello BA, Green LH, Grossman W, Cohn LH, Koster JK, Collins Jr. JJ. Hemodynamic determinants of prognosis of aortic valve replacement in critical aortic stenosis and advanced congestive heart failure. Circulation. 1980; 62:42-48.

32. Bonow RO. Management of chronic aortic regurgitation. N.Engl.J.Med. 1994; 331:736-737.

33. Carabello BA, Crawford FAJ. Valvular heart disease. N.Engl.J.Med. 1997; 337:32-41.

34. Cox JL, Sundt TM. The surgical management of atrial fibrillation. Annu.Rev.Med. 1997; 48:511-23.

35. Abascal VM, Wilkins GT, O'Shea JP, Choong CY, Palacios IF, Thomas JD, et al. Prediction of successful outcome in 130 patients undergoing percutaneous balloon mitral valvotomy. Circulation. 1990; 82:448-456.

36. Ben Farhat M, Ayari M, Maatouk F, Betbout F, Gamra H, Jarra M, Tiss M, Hammami S, Thaalbi R, Addad F. Percutaneous balloon versus surgical closed and open mitral commissurotomy: seven-year follow-up results of a randomized trial. Circulation. 1998; 97:245-250.

37. Bonow RO, Carabello B, de Leon AC, Edmunds LH, Jr., Fedderly BJ, Freed MD, Gaasch WH, McKay CR, Nishimura RA, O'Gara PT, O'Rourke RA, Rahimtoola SH, Ritchie JL, Cheitlin MD, Eagle KA, Gardner TJ, Garson A, Jr., Gibbons RJ, Russell RO, Ryan TJ, Smith SC, Jr. ACC/AHA Guidelines for the Management of Patients With Valvular Heart

Disease. Executive Summary. A report of the American College of Cardiology/American Heart Association Task Force on Practice Guidelines (Committee on Management of Patients With Valvular Heart Disease). J. Heart Valve Dis. 1998; 7:672-707.

38. Roudaut R, Labbe T, Lorient-Roudaut MF, Gosse P, Baudet E, Fontan F, et al. Mechanical cardiac valve thrombosis. Is fibrinolysis justified? Circulation. 1992; 86:II8-II5.

39. Lengyel M, Fuster V, Keltai M, Roudaut R, Schulte HD, Seward JB, Chesebro JH,Turpie AG. Guidelines for management of left-sided prosthetic valve thrombosis: a role for thrombolytic therapy. Consensus Conference on Prosthetic Valve Thrombosis. J. Am. Coll. Cardiol. 1997; 30:1521-1526.

40. Vaitkus PT, Kussmaul WG. Constrictive pericarditis versus restrictive cardiomyopathy: a reappraisal and update of diagnostic criteria. Am.Heart J. 1991; 122:1431-1441.

41. Guntheroth WG. Constrictive pericarditis versus restrictive cardiomyopathy. Circulation 1997; 95:542-543.

42. Masui T, Finck S, Higgins CB. Constrictive pericarditis and restrictive cardiomyopathy: evaluation with MR imaging. Radiology. 1992; 182:369-373.

43. McLaughlin VV, Genthner DE, Panella MM, Rich S. Reduction in pulmonary vascular resistance with long-term epoprostenol (prostacyclin) therapy in primary pulmonary hypertension. N.Engl.J.Med. 1998; 338:273-277.

CHAPTER 10 — OUTPATIENT THERAPY

1. Franciosa JA, Jordan RA, Wilen MM, Leddy CL. Minoxidil in patients with chronic left heart failure: contrasting hemodynamic and clinical effects in a controlled trial. Circulation. 1984; 70:63-68.

2. Pfeffer MA, Lamas GA, Vaughan DE, Parisi AF, Braunwald E. Effect of captopril on progressive ventricular dilatation after anterior myocardial infarction. N.Engl.J.Med. 1988; 319:80-86.

3. The SOLVD Investigators. Effect of enalapril on mortality and the development of heart failure in asymptomatic patients with reduced left ventricular ejection fractions. N.Engl.J.Med. 1992; 327:685-691.

4. Coats AJ, Exercise training for heart failure: coming of age. Circulation. 1999; 99:1138-1140.

5. Belardinelli R, Georgiou D, Cianci G, Purcaro A. Randomized, controlled trial of long-term moderate exercise training in chronic heart failure: effects on functional capacity, quality of life, and clinical outcome. Circulation. 1999; 99:1173-1182.

6. Hare DL, Ryan TM, Selig SE, Pellizzer AM, Wrigley TV, Krum H. Resistance exercise training increases muscle strength, endurance, and blood flow in patients with chronic heart failure. Am.J. Cardiol. 1999; 83:1674-1677, A7.

7. Lang RM, Borow KM, Neumann A, Feldman T. Adverse cardiac effects of acute alcohol ingestion in young adults. Ann.Intern.Med. 1985; 102:742-747.

8. Konstam MA, Dracup K, Baker DW. Heart failure: Evaluation and care of patients with left-ventricular systolic dysfunction. 1994; 11, US Department of Health and Human Services.

9. Krumholz HM, Butler J, Miller J, Vaccarino V, Williams CS, Mendes DLC, Seeman TE, Kasl SV, Berkman LF. Prognostic importance of emotional support for elderly patients hospitalized with heart failure. Circulation. 1998; 97:958-964.

10. Schiller E, Baker J. Return to work after a myocardial infarction: evaluation of planned rehabilitation and of a predictive rating scale. Med.J.Aust. 1976; 1:859-862.

11. Bar FW, Hoppener P, Diederiks J, Voken H, Bekkers J, Hoofd W. A Appels, HJ Wellins, Cardiac rehabilitation contributes to the restoration of leisure and social activities after myocardial infarction. J. Cardiopulm. Rehabil. 1992; 12:117-125.

12. Gutgesell HP, Gessner IH, Vetter VL, Yabek SM, Norton JBJ. Recreational and occupational recommendations for young patients with heart disease. A statement for physicians by the committee on congenital cardiac defects of the council on cardiovascular disease in the young, American Heart Association. Circulation. 1986; 74:1195A-1198A.

13. Fletcher G, Fernandez V. Screening and Evaluation of Patients for Exercise Training. In: Balady GJ, Pina I, editors. Exercise and heart failure. Armonk: Futura Publishing Company, Inc., 1997; 311–320.

14. Massie BM, Shah NB. Evolving trends in the epidemiologic factors of heart failure: rationale for preventive strategies and comprehensive disease management. Am.Heart J. 1997; 133:703-712.

15. Kostis JB, Davis BR, Cutler J, Grimm RH, Jr., Berge KG, Cohen JD, Lacy CR, Perry HM, Jr., Blaufox MD, Wassertheil-Smoller S, Black HR, Schron E, Berkson DM, Curb JD, Smith WM, McDonald R, Applegate WB. Prevention of heart failure by antihypertensive drug treatment in older persons with isolated systolic hypertension. SHEP Cooperative Research Group. JAMA 1997; 278:212-216.

16. Kjekshus J, Pedersen TH. Lowering of cholesterol with simvastatin may prevent development of heart failure in patients with coronary heart disease. Circulation. 1995; 282A.

17. Sueta CA, Chowdhury M, Boccuzzi SJ, Smith SCJ, Alexander CM, Londhe A, Lulla A, Simpson RJJ. Analysis of the degree of undertreatment of hyperlipidemia and congestive heart failure secondary to coronary artery disease. Am.J. Cardiol. 1999; 83:1303-1307.

18. Weber KT. Extracellular matrix remodeling in heart failure: a role for de novo angiotensin II generation. Circulation. 1997; 96:4065-4082.

19. Katz AM. The cardiomyopathy of overload: an unnatural growth response. Eur.Heart J. 1995; 16 (Suppl O):110-4.

20. Packer M. Consensus recommendations for the management of chronic heart failure. On behalf of the membership of the advisory council to improve outcomes nationwide in heart failure. Am. J. Cardiol. 1999; 83:1A-38A.

21. Pitt B, Zannad F, Remme WJ, Cody R, Castaigne A, Perez A, Palensky J, Wittes J. The effect of spironolactone on morbidity and mortality in patients with severe heart failure. N.Engl.J.Med. 1999; 341:709-717.

22. Brater DC. Diuretic therapy. N.Engl.J. Med. 1998; 339:387-395.

23. Brown NJ, Vaughan DE. Angiotensin-converting enzyme inhibitors. Circulation 1998; 97:1411-1420.

24. The SOLVD Investigators. Effect of enalapril on survival in patients with reduced left ventricular ejection fractions and congestive heart failure. N Engl J Med 1991; 325:293-302.

25. Packer M, Poole-Wilson PA, Armstrong PW, Cleland JG, Horowitz JD, Massie BM, Ryden L, Thygesen K, Uretsky BF. Comparative effects of low and high doses of the angiotensin-converting enzyme inhibitor, lisinopril, on morbidity and mortality in chronic heart failure. Circulation 1999; 100:2312-2318.

26. Pfeffer MA, Braunwald E, Moye LA, Basta L, Brown EJJ, Cuddy TE, et al. Effect of captopril on mortality and morbidity in patients with left ventricular dysfunction after myocardial infarction. Results of the survival and ventricular enlargement trial. The SAVE Investigators. N.Engl.J.Med. 1992; 327:669-677.

27. Gruppo Italiano per lo Studio della Sopravvivenza nell'infarto Miocardico. GISSI-3: effects of lisinopril and transdermal glyceryl trinitrate singly and together on 6-week mortality and ventricular function after acute myocardial infarction. Lancet.1994; 343:1115-1122.

28. ISIS-4 (Fourth International Study of Infarct Survival) Collaborative Group. ISIS-4: a randomised factorial trial assessing early oral captopril, oral mononitrate, and intravenous magnesium sulphate in 58,050 patients with suspected acute myocardial infarction. Lancet. 1995; 345:669-685.

29. M. St.John Sutton, Pfeffer MA, Plappert T, Rouleau JL, Moye LA, Dagenais GR, et al. Quantitative two-dimensional echocardiographic measurements are major predictors of adverse cardiovascular events after acute myocardial infarction. The protective effects of captopril. Circulation. 1994; 89:68-75.

30. Cohn JN, Johnson G, Ziesche S, Cobb F, Francis G, Tristani F, et al. A comparison of enalapril with hydralazine-isosorbide dinitrate in the treatment of chronic congestive heart failure. N.Engl.J.Med. 1991; 325:303-310.

31. The SOLVD Investigators. Effect of enalapril on survival in patients with reduced left ventricular ejection fractions and congestive heart failure. N.Engl.J.Med. 1991; 325:293-302.

32. The CONSENSUS Trial Study Group. Effects of enalapril on mortality in severe congestive heart failure. Results of the Cooperative North Scandinavian Enalapril Survival Study (CONSENSUS). N.Engl.J.Med. 1987; 316:1429-1435.

33. Brunner-La Rocca HP, Vaddadi G, Esler MD. Recent insight into therapy of congestive heart failure: focus on ACE inhibition and angiotensin-II antagonism. J. Am.Coll.Cardiol. 1999; 33:1163-1173.

34. Pitt B, Segal R, Martinez FA, Meurers G, Cowley AJ, Thomas I, et al. Randomised trial of losartan versus captopril in patients over 65 with heart failure (Evaluation of Losartan in the Elderly Study, ELITE). Lancet. 1997; 349:747-752.

35. Baruch L, Anand I, Cohen IS, Ziesche S, Judd D, Cohn JN. Augmented short- and long-term hemodynamic and hormonal effects of an angiotensin receptor blocker added to angiotensin converting enzyme inhibitor therapy in patients with heart failure. Circulation. 1999; 99:2658-2664.

36. Hamroff G, Katz SD, Mancini D, Blaufarb I, Bijou R, Patel R, Jondeau G, Olivari MT, Thomas S, Le Jemtel TH. Addition of angiotensin II receptor blockade to maximal angiotensin-converting enzyme inhibition improves exercise capacity in patients with severe congestive heart failure. Circulation. 1999; 99: 990-992.

37. Levine TB, Levine AB, Keteyian SJ, Narins B, Lesch M. Reverse remodeling in heart failure with intensification of vasodilator therapy. Clin.Cardiol. 1997; 20:697-702.

38. Cusick DA, Pfeifer PB, Quigg RJ. Effects of intravenous milrinone followed by titration of high-dose oral vasodilator therapy on clinical outcome and rehospitalization rates in patients with severe heart failure. Am. J. Cardiol. 1998; 82:1060-1065.

39. Cohn JN, Johnson G, Ziesche S, Cobb F, Francis G, Tristani F, Smith R, Dunkman WB, Loeb H, Wong M. A comparison of enalapril with hydralazine-isosorbide dinitrate in the treatment of chronic congestive heart failure. N.Engl.J.Med. 1991; 325:303-310.

40. Elkayam U, Johnson JV, Shotan A, Bokhari S, Solodky A, Canetti M, Wani OR, Karaalp IS. Double-blind, placebo-controlled study to evaluate the effect of organic nitrates in patients with chronic heart failure treated with angiotensin-converting enzyme inhibition. Circulation. 1999; 99:2652-2657.

41. Haude M, Steffen W, Erbel R, Meyer J. Sublingual administration of captopril versus nitroglycerin in patients with severe congestive heart failure. Int.J.Cardiol. 1990; 27:351-359.

42. Fifer MA, Colucci WS, Lorell BH, Jaski BE, Barry WH. Inotropic, vascular and neuroendocrine effects of nifedipine in heart failure: comparison with nitroprusside. J. Am. Coll. Cardiol. 1985; 5:731-737.

43. Muller JE, Morrison J, Stone PH, Rude RE, Rosner B, Roberts R, Pearle DL, Turi ZG, Schneider JF, Serfas DH. Nifedipine therapy for patients with threatened and acute myocardial infarction: a randomized, double-blind, placebo-controlled comparison. Circulation. 1984; 69:740-747.

44. Goldstein RE, Boccuzzi SJ, Cruess D, Nattel S. Diltiazem increases late-onset congestive heart failure in postinfarction patients with early reduction in ejection fraction. The Adverse Experience Committee; and the Multicenter Diltiazem Postinfarction Research Group. Circulation. 1991; 83:52-60.

45. Elkayam U. Calcium channel blockers in heart failure. Cardiology. 1998; 89 (Suppl 1):38-46.

46. Packer M, O'Connor CM, Ghali JK, Pressler ML, Carson PE, Belkin RN, et al. Effect of amlodipine on morbidity and mortality in severe chronic heart failure. Prospective Randomized Amlodipine Survival Evaluation Study Group. N.Engl.J.Med. 1996; 335:1107-1114.

47. O'Connor CM, Carson PE, Miller AB, Pressler ML, Belkin RN, Neuberg GW, Frid DJ, Cropp AB, Anderson S, Wertheimer JH, DeMets DL. Effect of amlodipine on mode of death among patients with advanced heart failure in the PRAISE trial. Prospective Randomized Amlodipine Survival Evaluation. Am.J. Cardiol. 1998; 82:881-887.

48. Cohn JN, Ziesche S, Smith R, Anand I, Dunkman WB, Loeb H, Cintron G, Boden W, Baruch L, Rochin P, Loss L. Effect of the calcium antagonist felodipine as supplementary vasodilator therapy in patients with chronic heart failure treated with enalapril: V-HeFT III. Vasodilator-Heart Failure Trial (V-HeFT) Study Group. Circulation. 1997; 96:856-863.

49. The Digitalis Investigation Group. The effect of digoxin on mortality and morbidity in patients with heart failure. N.Engl.J.Med. 1997; 336:525-533.

50. Ferguson DW, Berg WJ, Sanders JS, Roach PJ, Kempf JS, Kienzle MG. Sympathoinhibitory responses to digitalis glycosides in heart failure patients. Direct evidence from sympathetic neural recordings. Circulation. 1989; 80: 65-77.

51. Young JB, Gheorghiade M, Uretsky BF, Patterson JH, Adams KFJ. Superiority of "triple" drug therapy in heart failure: insights from the PROVED and RADIANCE trials. Prospective Randomized Study of Ventricular Function and Efficacy of Digoxin. Randomized Assessment of Digoxin and Inhibitors of Angiotensin-Converting Enzyme. J. Am.Coll.Cardiol. 1998; 32:686-692.

52. Waagstein F, Bristow MR, Swedberg K, Camerini F, Fowler MB, Silver MA, et al. Beneficial effects of metoprolol in idiopathic dilated cardiomyopathy. Metoprolol in Dilated Cardiomyopathy (MDC) Trial Study Group. Lancet. 1993; 342:1441-1446.

53. Effect of metoprolol CR/XL in chronic heart failure: Metoprolol CR/XL Randomised Intervention Trial in Congestive Heart Failure (MERIT-HF). Lancet. 1999; 353:2001-2007.

54. The CIBIS II Investigators and Committees. The Cardiac Insufficiency Bisoprolol Study II (CIBIS II): a randomised trial. Lancet 1999; 353:9-13.

55. Frishman WH. Carvedilol. N.Engl.J Med. 1998; 339:1759-1765.

56. Gilbert EM, Abraham WT, Olsen S, Hattler B, White M, Mealy P, et al. Comparative hemodynamic, left ventricular functional, and antiadrenergic effects of chronic treatment with metoprolol versus carvedilol in the failing heart. Circulation. 1996; 94:2817-2825.

57. Packer M, Bristow MR, Cohn JN, Colucci WS, Fowler MB, Gilbert EM, et al. The effect of carvedilol on morbidity and mortality in patients with chronic heart failure. U.S. Carvedilol Heart Failure Study Group. N.Engl.J.Med. 1996; 334:1349-1355.

58. Di Lenarda A, Sabbadini F, Salvatore L, Sinagra G, Mestroni L, Pinamonti B, Gregori D, Ciani F, Muzzi A, Klugmann S, Camerini F. Long-term effects of carvedilol in idiopathic dilated cardiomyopathy with persistent left ventricular dysfunction despite chronic metoprolol. The Heart-Muscle Disease Study Group. J. Am.Coll.Cardiol. 1999; 33:1926-1934.

59. Kukin ML, Kalman J, Charney RH, Levy DK, Buchholz-Varley C, Ocampo ON, Eng C. Prospective, randomized comparison of effect of long-term treatment with metoprolol or carvedilol on symptoms, exercise, ejection fraction, and oxidative stress in heart failure. Circulation. 1999; 99:2645-2651.

60. Hjalmarson A, Kneider M, Waagstein F. The role of beta-blockers in left ventricular dysfunction and heart failure. Drugs. 1997; 54:501-510.

61. Australia/New Zealand Heart Failure Research Collaborative Group. Randomised, placebo-controlled trial of carvedilol in patients with congestive heart failure due to ischaemic heart disease. Lancet. 1997; 349:375-380.

62. Lowes BD, Gill EA, Abraham WT, Larrain JR, Robertson AD, Bristow MR, Gilbert EM. Effects of carvedilol on left ventricular mass, chamber geometry, and mitral regurgitation in chronic heart failure. Am. J. Cardiol. 1999; 83:1201-1205.

63. Macdonald PS, Keogh AM, Aboyoun CL, Lund M, Amor R, McCaffrey DJ. Tolerability and efficacy of carvedilol in patients with New York Heart Association class IV heart failure. J. Am. Coll.Cardiol. 1999; 33:924-931.

64. Senni M, Redfield MM. Congestive heart failure in elderly patients. Mayo Clin.Proc.1997; 72:453-460.

65. Ruzumna P, Gheorghiade M, Bonow RO. Mechanisms and management of heart failure due to diastolic dysfunction. Curr.Opin.Cardiol. 1996; 11:269-275.

66. Vasan RS, Larson MG, Benjamin EJ, Evans JC, Reiss CK, Levy D. Congestive heart failure in subjects with normal versus reduced left ventricular ejection fraction: prevalence and mortality in a population- based cohort. J. Am.Coll.Cardiol. 1999; 33:1948-1955.

67. Nishimura RA, Tajik AJ. Evaluation of diastolic filling of left ventricle in health and disease: Doppler echocardiography is the clinician's Rosetta Stone. J.Am.Coll.Cardiol. 1997; 30:8-18.

68. Neaton JD, Grimm RHJ, Prineas RJ, Stamler J, Grandits GA, Elmer PJ, et al. Treatment of mild hypertension study. Final results. Treatment of Mild Hypertension Study Research Group. JAMA. 1993; 270:713-724.

69. Spirito P, Seidman CE, McKenna WJ, Maron BJ. The management of hypertrophic cardi-omyopathy. N.Engl.J.Med. 1997; 336:775-785.

70. Nishimura RA, Trusty JM, Hayes DL, Ilstrup DM, Larson DR, Hayes SN, et al. Dual-chamber pacing for hypertrophic cardiomyopathy: a randomized, double-blind, crossover trial. J.Am.Coll.Cardiol. 1997; 29:435-441.

71. Spirito P, Seidman CE, McKenna WJ, Maron BJ. The management of hypertrophic cardi-omyopathy. N.Engl.J.Med. 1997; 336:775-785.

72. Maron BJ , Nishimura RA, McKenna WJ, Rakowski H, Josephson ME, Kieval RS. Assessment of permanent dual-chamber pacing as a treatment for drug- refractory symptomatic patients with obstructive hypertrophic cardiomyopathy. A randomized, double-blind, cross-over study (M-PATHY). Circulation. 1999; 99:2927-2933.

73. Ommen SR, Nishimura RA, Squires RW, Schaff HV, Danielson GK , Tajik AJ. Comparison of dual-chamber pacing versus septal myectomy for the treatment of patients with hypertropic obstructive cardiomyopathy: a comparison of objective hemodynamic and exercise end points. J. Am.Coll.Cardiol. 1999; 34:191-196.

74. Sigwart U. Non-surgical myocardial reduction for hypertrophic obstructive cardiomyopathy. Lancet. 1995; 346:211-214.

75. Seggewiss H, Gleichmann U, Faber L, Fassbender D, Schmidt HK, Strick S. Percutaneous transluminal septal myocardial ablation in hypertrophic obstructive cardiomyopathy: acute results and 3-month follow-up in 25 patients. J.Am.Coll.Cardiol. 1998; 31:252-258.

76. Primo J, Geelen P, Brugada J, Filho AL, Mont L, Wellens F, Valentino M, Brugada P. Hyper-trophic cardiomyopathy: role of the implantable cardioverter-defibrillator. J.Am.Coll.Cardiol. 1998; 31:1081-1085.

77. Psaty BM, Manolio TA, Kuller LH, Kronmal RA, Cushman M, Fried LP, White R, Furberg CD, Rautaharju PM. Incidence of and risk factors for atrial fibrillation in older adults. Circu-lation. 1997; 96:2455-2461.

78. Waktare JE, Camm AJ. Acute treatment of atrial fibrillation: why and when to maintain sinus rhythm. Am.J.Cardiol. 1998; 8:3C-15C.

79. Stevenson WG, Stevenson LW. Atrial fibrillation in heart failure. N.Engl.J Med. 1999; 341:910-911.

80. Brodsky MA, Allen BJ, Capparelli EV, Luckett CR, Morton R, Henry WL. Factors determining maintenance of sinus rhythm after chronic atrial fibrillation with left atrial dilatation. Am.J.Cardiol. 1989; 63:1065-1068.

81. Brignole M, Menozzi C, Gianfranchi L, Musso G, Mureddu R, Bottoni N and Lolli G. Assessment of atrioventricular junction ablation and VVIR pacemaker versus pharmacological treatment in patients with heart failure and chronic atrial fibrillation: a randomized, controlled study. Circulation. 1998; 98:953-960.

82. Goodman, Gilman. The pharmacological basis of therapeutics. 8 ed. Philadelphia: McGraw Hill, 1990; 866-869.

83. Kaye DM, Dart AM, Jennings GL , Esler MD. Antiadrenergic effect of chronic amiodarone therapy in human heart failure. J. Am.Coll.Cardiol. 1999; 33:1553-1559.

84. Boutitie F, Boissel JP, Connolly SJ, Camm AJ, Cairns JA, Julian DG, Gent M, Janse MJ, Dorian P, Frangin G. Amiodarone interaction with beta-blockers: analysis of the merged EMIAT (European Myocardial Infarct Amiodarone Trial) and CAMIAT (Canadian Amiodarone Myocardial Infarction Trial) databases. The EMIAT and CAMIAT Investigators. Circulation. 1999; 99:2268-2275.

85. The Antiarrhythmics versus Implantable Defibrillators (AVID) Investigators. A comparison of antiarrhythmic-drug therapy with implantable defibrillators in patients resuscitated from near-fatal ventricular arrhythmias. N.Engl.J.Med. 1997; 337:1576-1583.

86. Moss AJ, Hall WJ, Cannom DS, Daubert JP, Higgins SL, Klein H, et al. Improved survival with an implanted defibrillator in patients with coronary disease at high risk for ventricular arrhythmia. Multicenter Automatic Defibrillator Implantation Trial Investigators. N.Engl.J.Med. 1996; 335:1933-1940.

87. Al-Khadra AS, Salem DN, Rand WM, Udelson JE, Smith JJ, Konstam MA. Warfarin anticoagulation and survival: a cohort analysis from the Studies of Left Ventricular Dysfunction. J.Am.Coll.Cardiol. 1998; 31:749-753.

88. Rich MW, Freedland KE. Effect of DRGs on three-month readmission rate of geriatric patients with congestive heart failure. Am.J.Public Health 1988; 78:680-682.

89. Shah NB, Der E, Ruggerio C, Heidenreich PA, Massie BM. Prevention of hospitalizations for heart failure with an interactive home monitoring program. Am.Heart J. 1998;135:373-378.

90. Fonarow GC, Stevenson LW, Walden JA, Livingston NA, Steimle AE, Hamilton MA, et al. Impact of a comprehensive heart failure management program on hospital readmission and functional status of patients with advanced heart failure. J.Am.Coll.Cardiol. 1997; 30:725-732.

91. Mancini DM, Eisen H, Kussmaul W, Mull R, Edmunds LHG, Wilson JR. Value of peak exercise oxygen consumption for optimal timing of cardiac transplantation in ambulatory patients with heart failure. Circulation. 1991; 83:778-786.

92. Stelken AM, Younis LT, Jennison SH, Miller DD, Miller LW, Shaw LJ, Kargl D, Chaitman BR. Prognostic value of cardiopulmonary exercise testing using percent achieved of predicted peak oxygen uptake for patients with ishemic and dilated cardiomyopathy. J.Am.Coll.Cardiol. 1996; 27:345-352.

93. Anker SD, Ponikowski P, Varney S, Chua TP, Clark AL, Webb-Peploe KM, Harrington D, Kox WJ, Poole-Wilson PA, Coats AJ. Wasting as independent risk factor for mortality in chronic heart failure. Lancet. 1997; 349:1050-1053.

94. Fletcher G, Balady G, Froelicher VF and et al. Exercise Standards. A statement for healthcare professionals from the American Heart Association.Circulation. 1995; 91:580.

95. Kobashigawa JA. Mycophenolate mofetil in cardiac transplantation. Curr.Opin.Cardiol. 1998; 13:117-121.

96. Mentzer RMJ, Jahania MS, Lasley RD. Tacrolimus as a rescue immunosuppressant after heart and lung transplantation. The U.S. Multicenter FK506 Study Group. Transplantation. 1998; 65:109-113.

97. Hosenpud JD, Bennett LE, Keck BM, Fiol B, Novick RJ. The registry of the international society for heart and lung transplantation: fourteenth official report—1997. J.Heart Lung Transplant. 1997; 16:691-712.

CHAPTER 11 — INPATIENT THERAPY

1. Feenstra J, Grobbee DE, Remme WJ, Stricker BH. Drug-induced heart failure. J. Am.Coll.Cardiol. 1999; 33:1152-1162.

2. Konstam MA, Dracup K, Baker DW. Heart failure: Evaluation and care of patients with left-ventricular systolic dysfunction. US Department of Health and Human Services 1994; 11.

3. Comroe JH. Exploring the heart: discoveries in heart disease and high blood pressure. New York: Norton, 1983; 123–125.

4. Hostetter TH, Manske CL, Paller MS. Continuous hemofiltration. N.Engl.J.Med. 1997; 337:712-713.

5. Forni LG, Hilton PJ. Continuous hemofiltration in the treatment of acute renal failure. N.Engl.J.Med. 1997; 336:1303-1309.

6. Stegmayr BG, Banga R, Lundberg L, Wikdahl AM, Plum-Wirell M. PD treatment for severe congestive heart failure. Perit.Dial.Int. 1996; 16 (Suppl 1):S231-235.

7. Thadani U. Nitrate tolerance, rebound, and their clinical relevance in stable angina pectoris, unstable angina, and heart failure. Cardiovasc.Drugs Ther. 1997; 10:735-742.

8. Breisblatt WM, Navratil DL, Burns MJ, Spaccavento LJ. Comparable effects of intravenous nitroglycerin and intravenous nitroprusside in acute ischemia. Am.Heart J. 1988; 116:465-472.

9. Mann T, Cohn PF, Holman LB, Green LH, Markis JE, Phillips DA. Effect of nitroprusside on regional myocardial blood flow in coronary artery disease. Results in 25 patients and comparison with nitroglycerin. Circulation. 1978; 57:732-738.

10. Jaski BE, Fifer MA, Wright RF, Braunwald E, Colucci WS. Positive inotropic and vasodilator actions of milrinone in patients with severe congestive heart failure. Dose-response relationships and comparison to nitroprusside. J.Clin.Invest. 1985; 75:643-649.

11. Leier CV, Unverferth DV. Drugs five years later. Dobutamine. Ann.Intern.Med. 1983; 99:490-496.

12. Goldberg LI. Dopamine—clinical uses of an endogenous catecholamine. N.Engl.J.Med. 1974; 291:707-710.

13. Farmer JB. Indirect sympathomimetic actions of dopamine. J.Pharm.Pharmacol. 1966; 18:261-262.

14. Colucci WS, Wright RF, Jaski BE, Fifer MA, Braunwald E. Milrinone and dobutamine in severe heart failure: differing hemodynamic effects and individual patient responsiveness. Circulation. 1986; 73:III175-III183.

15. Loeb HS, Bredakis J, Gunner RM. Superiority of dobutamine over dopamine for augmentation of cardiac output in patients with chronic low output cardiac failure. Circulation. 1977; 55:375-378.

16. Monrad ES, Baim DS, Smith HS, Lanoue AS. Milrinone, dobutamine, and nitroprusside: comparative effects on hemodynamics and myocardial energetics in patients with severe congestive heart failure. Circulation. 1986; 73:III168-III174.

17. Leier CV, Heban PT, Huss P, Bush CA, Lewis RP. Comparative systemic and regional hemodynamic effects of dopamine and dobutamine in patients with cardiomyopathic heart failure. Circulation. 1978; 58:466-475.

18. Mills RM, LeJemtel TH, Horton DP, Liang C, Lang R, Silver MA, Lui C, Chatterjee K. Sustained hemodynamic effects of an infusion of nesiritide (human b- type natriuretic peptide) in heart failure: a randomized, double-blind, placebo-controlled clinical trial. Natrecor Study Group. J. Am.Coll.Cardiol. 1999; 34:155-162.

19. Leier CV, Binkley PF. Parenteral inotropic support for advanced congestive heart failure. Prog.Cardiovasc.Dis. 1998; 41:207-224.

20. Grines CL, Browne KF, Marco J, Rothbaum D, Stone GW, O'Keefe J, et al. A comparison of immediate angioplasty with thrombolytic therapy for acute myocardial infarction. The Primary Angioplasty in Myocardial Infarction Study Group. N.Engl.J.Med. 1993; 328:673-679.

21. Stone GW, Brodie BR, Griffin JJ, Morice MC, Costantini C, St, et al. Prospective, multicenter study of the safety and feasibility of primary stenting in acute myocardial infarction: in-hospital and 30-day results of the PAMI stent pilot trial. Primary Angioplasty in Myocardial Infarction Stent Pilot Trial Investigators. J.Am.Coll.Cardiol. 1998; 31:23-30.

22. Jaski BE, Cohen JD, Trausch J, Marsh DG, Bail GR, Overlie PA, Skowronski EW, Smith SC Jr. Outcome of urgent percutaneous transluminal coronary angioplasty in acute myocardial infarction: comparison of single-vessel versus multivessel coronary artery disease. Am.Heart J. 1992; 124:1427-1433.

23. Mills RM, Pepine CJ. Heart failure secondary to coronary artery disease. In: Hosenpud JD, Greenberg BH. Congestive heart failure: Pathophysiology, diagnosis, and comprehensive approach to mangement. New York: Springer-Verlag, 1994;185.

24. Page DL, Caulfield JB, Kastor JA, DeSanctis RW, Sanders CA. Myocardial changes associated with cardiogenic shock. N.Engl.J.Med. 1971; 285:133-137.

25. Holmes DRJ, Bates ER, Kleiman NS, Sadowski Z, Horgan JH, Morris DC, Califf RM, Berger PB, Topol EJ. Contemporary reperfusion therapy for cardiogenic shock: the GUSTO-I trial experience. The GUSTO-I Investigators. Global Utilization of Streptokinase and Tissue Plasminogen Activator for Occluded Coronary Arteries. J.Am.Coll.Cardiol. 1995; 26:668-674.

26. Goldberg RJ, Samad NA, Yarzebski Y, Gurwitz J, Bigelow C, Gore JM. Temporal trends in cardiogenic shock complicating acute myocardial infarction. N.Engl.J. Med. 1999; 340:1162-1168.

27. Reichman RT, Joyo CI, Dembitsky WP, Griffith LD, Adamson RM, Daily PO, Overlie PA, Smith, SC Jr., Jaski BE. Improved patient survival after cardiac arrest using a cardiopulmonary support system. Ann.Thorac.Surg. 1990; 49:101-104.

28. Dembitsky WP, Moore CH, Holman WL, Jaski BE, Moreno-Cabral RJ, Adamson RM, Daily PO, Moreno-Cabral CE. Successful mechanical circulatory support for noncoronary shock. J.Heart Lung Transplant. 1992; 11:129-135.

29. Hochman J, Sleeper LA, Webb JG, Sanborn TA, White HD, Talley JD, Buller CE, Jacobs AK, Slater JN, Col J, McKinlya SM, LeJemtel TH, Picard MH, Menegus MA, Boland J, Dzavik V, Thompson CR, Wong SC, Steingart R, Forman R, Aylward PE, Godfrey E and Desvigne-Nickens P, for the SHOCK investigators. Early revascularization in acute myocardial infarction complicated by cardiogenic shock. N.Engl.J. Med. 1999; 341:625-634.

30. Grauer K. ACLS. 3 ed. St. Lous: Mosby, 1993.

31. Jaski BE, Branch KR. Supported circulation in the cardiac catheterization laboratory. In: Peterson KL, Nicod P, editors. Cardiac catheterization: Methods, diagnosis, and therapy. Philadelphia: WB Saunders, 1997; 545-564.

32. Quaal S. Conventional timing using the arterial pressure waveform. In: Quaal S, editor. Comprehensive intra-aortic balloon counterpulsation. St. Louis: Mosby, 1993;246-259.

33. Moulopoulos SD, Topaz S, Kolff WJ. Diastolic balloon pumping (with carbon dioxide) in the aorta: A mechanical assistance to the failing circulation. Am.Heart J. 1962; 63:669-675.

34. Gewirtz H, Ohley W, Williams DO, Sun Y, Most AS. Effect of intraaortic balloon counter pulsation on regional myocardial blood flow and oxygen consumption in the presence of coronary artery stenosis: observations in an awake animal model. Am.J.Cardiol. 1982; 50:829-837.

35. Leinbach RC, Buckley MJ, Austen WG, Petschek HE, Kantrowitz AR, Sanders CA. Effects of intra-aortic balloon pumping on coronary flow and metabolism in man. Circulation. 1971; 43:I77-I81.

36. Amsterdam ES, Awan NA, Lee G, et al. Intra-aortic balloon counterpulsation: Rationale, application, and results. In: Rackley CE, ed. Critical Care Cardiology. Philadelphia: F.A. Davis, 1981.

37. Cadwell CA, Tyson G. Real timing. In: Quaal S, editor. Comprehensive intra-aortic balloon counterpulsation. St. Louis: Mosby, 1993; 281-294.
38. Clements SDJ, Story WE, Hurst JW, Craver JM, Jones EL. Ruptured papillary muscle, a complication of myocardial infarction: clinical presentation, diagnosis, and treatment. Clin.Cardiol. 1985; 8:93-103.
39. Bolooki H. Emergency cardiac procedures in patients in cardiogenic shock due to complications of coronary artery disease. Circulation. 1989; 79:1137-1148.
40. Murphy DA, Craver JM, Jones EL, Curling PE, Guyton RA, King SB, et al. Surgical management of acute myocardial ischemia following percutaneous transluminal coronary angioplasty. Role of the intra-aortic balloon pump. J.Thorac.Cardiovasc.Surg. 1984; 87:332-339.
41. Chaudary S, Jaski BE. Fulminant mumps myocarditis. Ann.Intern.Med. 1989; 110:569-570.
42. Mackenzie DJ, Wagner WH, Kulber DA, Treiman RL, Cossman DV, Foran RF, Cohen JL, Levin PM. Vascular complications of the intra-aortic balloon pump. Am.J.Surg. 1992; 164:517-521.
43. Comroe JH. Exploring the heart: discoveries in heart disease and high blood pressure. New York: Norton, 1983; 15-19, 26-27, 30-36.
44. Dembitsky WP, Moreno-Cabral RJ, Adamson RM, Daily PO. Emergency resuscitation using portable extracorporeal membrane oxygenation. Ann.Thorac.Surg. 1993; 55:304-309.
45. Jaski BE, McClendon PS, Branch KR, Favrot LK, Smith SCJ, Lamphere J, et al. Antero grade perfusion in acute limb ischemia secondary to vascular occlusive cardiopulmonary support. Cathet.Cardiovasc.Diagn. 1995; 35:373-376.
46. Willms DC, Atkins PJ, Dembitsky WP, Jaski BE, Gocka I. Analysis of clinical trends in a program of emergent ECLS for cardiovascular collapse. ASAIO.J. 1997; 43:65-68.
47. Jaski BE, Lingle RJ, Overlie P, Favrot LK, Willms DC, Dembitsky WP. Long term survival with use of percutaneous cardiopulmonary support in patients presenting with acute myocardial infarction and cardiovascular collapse. ASAIO J. 1999; 45:615-618.
48. Vogel RA, Shawl F, Tommaso C, O'Neill W, Overlie P, O'Toole J, Vandormael M, Topol E, Tabari KK, Vogel J. Initial report of the National Registry of Elective Cardiopulmonary Bypass Supported Coronary Angioplasty. J.Am.Coll.Cardiol. 1990; 15:23-29.
49. Jaski BE, Kim J, Maly RS, Branch KR, Adamson R, Favrot LK, et al. Effects of exercise during long-term support with a left ventricular assist device. Results of the experience with left ventricular assist device with exercise (EVADE) pilot trial. Circulation. 1997; 95:2401-2406.
50. Jaski BE, Lingle RJ, Kim J, Branch KR, Goldsmith RL, Johnson MR, Lahpor J, Icenogle T, Pina I, Adamson R, Favrot LK, Dembitsky W for The EVADE Investigator Group. A multicenter prospective paired comparison of functional capacity in patients with end-stage heart failure following implantation of a left ventricular assist device versus heart transplantation. J. Heart Lung Transplant 1999; 18:1031-1040.
51. Goldstein DJ, Oz MC, Rose EA. Implantable left ventricular assist devices. N.Engl.J. Med. 1998; 339:1522-1533 .
52. DiSesa VJ. Cardiac xenotransplantation. Ann.Thorac.Surg. 1997; 64:1858-1865.
53. Cohn JN, Bristow MR, Chien KR, Colucci WS, Frazier OH, Leinwand LA, et al. Report of the National Heart, Lung, and Blood Institute special emphasis panel on heart failure research. Circulation. 1997; 95:766-770.

Appendix

Longitudinal vs. Transmural Pressure

Pressure is a force per unit area. It is a property of a fluid or gas that pushes outward uniformly in all directions. Pressure within a tube can result in flow that is proportional to the *longitudinal* (P_1 - P_2) difference in pressure along the tube. In addition, flow in a straight tube is highly dependent on the diameter of the tube and is proportional to $1/(\text{radius of tube})^4$.

VESSEL OR CHAMBER DISTENTION

Pressure also distends an elastic blood vessel or cardiac chamber. In general, a volume will increase within elastic walls to the *transmural* pressure difference, P_1 - P_0.

This explains why arterial proportional pulse pressue (SBP-DBP/SBP) is a good predictor of stroke volume and, therefore, cardiac index (see page 30).

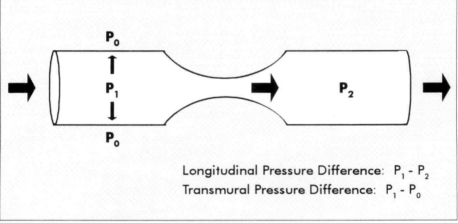

Longitudinal Pressure Difference: P_1 - P_2

Transmural Pressure Difference: P_1 - P_0

Figure A-1. *Longitudinal vs. Transmural Pressure: longitudinal pressure determines* **flow;** *whereas transmural pressure determines* **volume.**

Basic Concept of Wall Tension in Elastic Materials (Force/Length) : LaPlace's Law

It is often useful to estimate forces in materials that generate a pressure within a chamber such as the heart. In a thin-walled sphere filled with a fluid under pressure (P), there is a force per unit length of the circumference that keeps the chamber from exploding. Tension (T) is analogous to wall stress (σ — force/area) in a thick-walled sphere like the heart. The total force pulling each hemisphere apart is equal to the product of the pressure (P) and the projected area of the hemisphere. This must be supported by the edge between the two hemispheres of length $2\Pi r$. Notice that the required tension within the material increases in proportion to the increase in radius of the sphere.

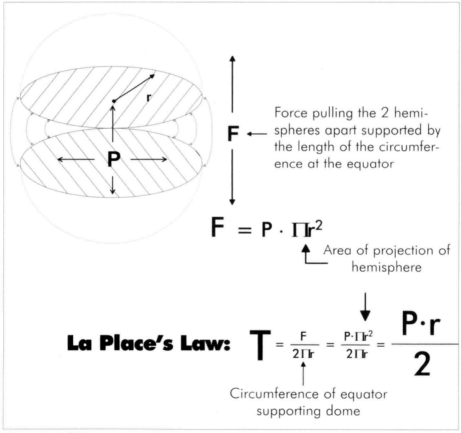

Force pulling the 2 hemi-
$F \longleftarrow$ spheres apart supported by
the length of the circumfer-
ence at the equator

$$F = P \cdot \Pi r^2$$

Area of projection of
hemisphere

La Place's Law: $\quad T = \dfrac{F}{2\Pi r} = \dfrac{P \cdot \Pi r^2}{2\Pi r} = \dfrac{P \cdot r}{2}$

Circumference of equator
supporting dome

Figure A-2. Wall tension in elastic materials. In heart failure the increased size of the left ventricular chamber leads to a higher afterload for any given systolic pressure.

Basic Concept of Wall Stress in Elastic Materials: Hooke's Law

Hooke's law states that in "elastic" materials the force per unit area (stress, σ) is proportional to the stretch or compression (ΔL) divided by the total length (L_o) of multiplied by a stretch factor, E.

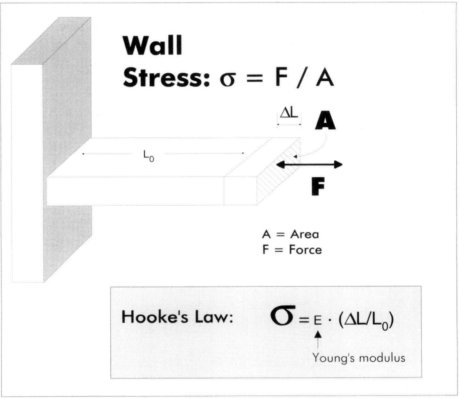

Wall
Stress: $\sigma = F / A$

ΔL **A**

L_0

F

A = Area
F = Force

Hooke's Law: $\sigma = E \cdot (\Delta L/L_0)$

Young's modulus

Figure A-3. *Wall stress in elastic materials.*

STRESS DIFFERS FROM PRESSURE

Stress differs from pressure, which is also a force /area. Any given value of stress deforms a material *along a single direction* and in general varies across the material being deformed — it is a vector quantity. Any given value of pressure (for example, within the left ventricular chamber) is a *property* of the contained fluid or gas, pushing *outward uniformly in all directions* — it is a scalar quantity.

Summary of Clinical Trials of Therapy for Heart Failure

TRIALS

	Design	Results
DIGOXIN TRIALS		
DIG: Digitalis Investigation Group (NEJM 1997;336:525)	6800 patients with heart failure, sinus rhythm, and EF < 45% randomized to digoxin or placebo.	No difference in overall mortality. Lower incidence of death or hospitalization due to worsening heart failure with digoxin (27% vs 35%).
RADIANCE: Randomized Assessment of Digoxin or Inhibitors of the Angiotensin-Converting Enzyme (NEJM 1993;329:1)	178 patients in sinus rhythm, Class II-III heart failure, EF < 35%, and stable on digoxin, diuretics and ACE inhibitor randomized to continue receiving digoxin or digoxin withdrawal for 12 wks.	Worsening heart failure necessitating withdrawal from study occurred more often in placebo group (25%) than those maintained on digoxin (5%). Ventricular function also deteriorated when digoxin was withdrawn.
PROVED: Prospective Randomized study of Ventricular failure and the Efficacy of Digoxin (JACC 1993;22:955)	88 patients with mild-moderate CHF receiving digoxin (median dose 0.37 mg/d) and diuretics randomized to continue receiving digoxin or digoxin withdrawal for 12 wks.	Patients withdrawn from digoxin had decreased exercise tolerance, deterioration in ventricular function, and more frequent progression of heart failure symptoms (39% vs 19%).
ACE INHIBITOR TRIALS	Design	Results
V-HeFT II: Veteran's Administration Heart Failure Trial II. (NEJM 1991;325:303)	804 men with same entry criteria as V-HeFT I trial randomized to hydralazine/isordil combination (75 mg + 40 mg qid) or enalapril (10 mg bid).	At 2 years, there was decreased mortality in enalapril compared to hydralazine/isordil group (18% vs 28.2%). Mortality benefit due to a reduction in sudden cardiac death.
ATLAS: Assessment of Treatment with Lisinopril and Survival (Circulation 1999; 100:2312-2318)	Patients with moderate-severe CHF randomized to low dose lisinopril (2.5-5 mg/d) or high dose lisinopril (32.5-5 mg/d).	Lower incidence of adverse events with high dose lisinopril.
SOLVD Treatment Trial: Studies of Left Ventricular Dysfunction (NEJM 1991;325:293)	2569 patients with chronic heart failure with EF < 35% not receiving drug treatment for heart failure randomized to enalapril (2.5-10 mg bid) or placebo.	Lower incidence of death or hospitalization due to heart failure in enalapril group compared to placebo (48% vs 57%).
SOLVD Prevention Trial: Studies of Left Ventricular Dysfunction (NEJM 1992;327:685)	4,228 asymptomatic patients with EF < 35% not receiving drug treatment for heart failure randomized to enalapril (2.5-20 mg/d) or placebo.	At average follow-up of 37 months, combined endpoint of death or heart failure was lower in enalapril group compared to placebo (30% vs 39%). Fewer hospitalizations for enalapril group (21% vs 25% for placebo).

A II RECEPTOR BLOCKER TRIALS	Design	Results
ELITE: Evaluation of Losartan in the Elderly (Lancet 1997;349:747)	722 patients with Class II-IV CHF and EF < 40% randomized to captopril (6.25-50 mg tid) plus placebo or losartan (12.5-50 mg/d) plus placebo.	Lower mortality (4.8% vs 8.7%), hospitalization rate (22% vs 30%), and side effects with losartan.
ELITE II : Evaluation of Losartan in the Elderly II (Circulation 1999; 100 (Supl I):I-782)	Preliminary report of 3,152 patients with Class II-IV CHF and EF< 40% randomized to captopril (12.5-50 mg tid) or losartan (12.5-50 mg/d) plus placebo.	All cause mortality shows no statistically significant difference (captopril 16% vs. losartan 18%).

β-BLOCKER TRIALS	Design	Results
Carvedilol Heart Failure Study (NEJM 1996;334:1349)	1094 patients with symptomatic heart failure for > 3 months and EF < 35% receiving diuretics and ACE inhibitors randomized to carvedilol (12.5-50 mg bid) or placebo.	Lower mortality (3.2% vs 7.8%), and hospitalization due to cardiovascular causes (14% vs 20%) with carvedilol.
Australia/New Zealand Heart Failure Research Collaborative Group (Lancet 1997;349:375)	415 patients with Class II-III CHF and EF < 45% randomized to carvedilol (6.25-25 mg bid) or placebo.	Increase in EF (5.3%), and decrease mortality or hospitalization with carvedilol (104 vs 131).
MERIT-HF: Metoprolol CR/XL Randomised Intervention Trial in Congestive Heart Failure (Lancet 1999; 353:2001-2007)	3991 patients with Class II-IV CHF and ejection fraction ≤ 40 randomized to metoprolol CR/XL with a target dose of 200 mg q.d. or placebo.	Lower all-cause mortality in the metoprolol CR/XL group than in the placebo group (7.2% vs 11.0%). Fewer sudden deaths and deaths from worsening heart failure.
CIBIS-II : The Cardiac Insufficiency Bisoprolol Study II (Lancet 1999; 353:9-13)	2647 patients with Class III or IV CHF, with left-ventricular ejection fraction ≤ 35% receiving standard therapy with diuretics and ACE inhibitors randomized to bisoprolol 1.25 mg/day or placebo daily, the drug was increased to a maximum of 10 mg/day.	Lower all-cause mortality with bisoprolol than placebo (11.8% vs 17.3%). Fewer sudden deaths among patients on bisoprolol than in those on placebo. Treatment effects independent of the severity or cause of heart failure. Efficacy not proven in patients wi

CALCIUM BLOCKER TRIALS	Design	Results
VHeFT III: Veteran's Administration Heart Failure Trial III (Circulation 1997;856:863)	450 patients with CHF and EF < 45% receiving diuretics and enalapril randomized to felodipine (5 mg bid) or placebo.	Prevention of worsening exercise tolerance and worsening quality of life with felodipine.
PRAISE: Prospective Randomized Amlodipine Survival Evaluation trial (NEJM 1996;335:1107)	1153 patients with Class IIIB -IV CHF and EF < 30% receiving digoxin, diuretics, and ACE inhibitor inhibitors randomized to amlodipine (5 mg/d for 14 d then 10 mg/d) or placebo.	Lower mortality in patients with non-ischemic CMP with amlodipine (28% vs 37%), but no difference in patients with CAD.

TRIALS OF OTHER AGENTS	Design	Results
AVID: Antiarrhythmics versus Implantable Defibrillators trial (NEJM 1997;337:1576)	1016 patients with near-fatal ventricular fibrillation or sustained ventricular tachycardia and EF < 40% randomized to receive implantable cardioverter-defibrillator or class III antiarrhythmic drugs.	Higher survival at 3 years with implantable defibrillator (75% vs 64%).
MADIT: The Multicenter Automatic Defibrillator Implantation Trial (NEJM 1996;335:1933)	196 patients with MI > 3 weeks before entry, episode of asymptomatic, nonsustained ventricular tachycardia, and EF<35% randomized to implantation of defibrillator or medical therapy.	Increased survival with implantation of defibrillator (15 deaths vs 39 deaths).
CHF-STAT: Survival Trial of Antiarrhythmic Therapy (JACC 1997;514:517)	674 patients with CHF and EF < 40% receiving vasodilator therapy randomized to amiodarone (800 mg/d for 14d, 400 mg/d for 50 weeks, 300 mg/d thereafter) or placebo.	No significant difference in survival after 1 and 2 years between groups.
GESICA: Group Study of Heart Failure in Argentina (Lancet 1994;344:493)	516 patients with Class II-IV and EF < 35% randomized to amiodarone (600 mg/d for 14 d then 300 mg/d for 2 years) or placebo.	Lower mortality with low-dose amiodarone (34% vs 41%).
V-HeFT I: Veteran' Administration Heart Failure Trial I (NEJM 1986;314:1547)	642 men with mild-moderate heart failure receiving digoxin and diuretics randomized to placebo, prazosin (5 mg qid), or combination therapy with hydralazine (max 75 mg qid) and isordil (max 40 mg qid).	2-year mortality lower in hydralazine/isordil group compared to placebo (26% vs 34%), as well as improved ventricular function. Prazosin not different from placebo.
RALES: Randomized Aldactone Evaluation Study Investigators (NEJM 1999; 341:709-717)	1663 patients with severe heart failure and LV ejection fraction ≤ 35% and being treated with an ACE inhibitor, a loop diuretic, and in most cases digoxin randomized to 25 mg of spironolactone daily and to placebo.	30% reduction in the risk of death in the spironolactone group due to a lower risk of death from progressive heart failure and sudden death. Frequency of hospitalization for worsening heart failure was 35% lower in the spironolactone group than in the placebo group. Side effects: Gynecomastia in 10% of men.

Chapter Quiz Solutions

CHAPTER 1 QUIZ- POPULATION

1. Each year approximately _____ people have a new onset of heart failure in the US.
   c) 400,000

2. Due to recent advances in the treatment of cardiovascular disease, the age-related death rate of heart failure has significantly declined over the past decade.
   b) False

3. From 1950 to1970, _____ was the major etiology of heart failure. With improvements in the treatment of this etiologic factor, _____ is now the dominant cause of heart failure in the US.
   b) hypertension; coronary artery disease

4. The severity of hypertension predicts the occurrence of heart failure and can lead to heart failure on the basis of systolic or diastolic dysfunction.
   a) True

5. Although the incidence of heart failure is greater in women than in men, men survive longer with heart failure, leading to a similar prevalence in any given age group of heart failure between men and women.
   b) False

6. Heart failure costs the US an estimated _____ dollars annually.
   c) 38 billion

CHAPTER 2 QUIZ- INDIVIDUAL

1. Paroxysomal nocturnal dyspnea is usually described as:
   c) dyspnea which appears suddenly at night, usually waking the patient after an hour or two of sleep

2. Complete this analogy: Forward heart failure: Inadequate tissue perfusion :: Backward heart failure: _____
   a) Pulmonary congestion

3. Some common manifestations of left heart failure include dyspnea, pulmonary congestion, and pulmonary edema. Right heart failure usually leads to
   d) none of the above

4. According to the Framingham Heart Study, all of the following are considered a 'major' criteria for heart failure except:
   a) night cough

5. All of the following cardiac events lead to an increase in symptoms in the patients with heart failure except:
   c) absent abdominojugular reflux

CHAPTER 2 QUIZ- INDIVIDUAL CON'T

6. In patients with known advanced heart failure, orthopnea was a more sensitive predictor of pulmonary capillary wedge pressure than other history or physical exam findings.
    a) True

7. In the patient with chronic heart failure, a physical exam can be free of findings of lung congestion despite a markedly elevated pulmonary capillary wedge pressure.
    a) True

CHAPTER 3 QUIZ- CIRCULATION

1. A patient has high filling pressures, depressed cardiac index, and normal blood pressure. The patient most likely has which type of heart failure?
    b) decompensated heart failure

2. Check (√) the value(s) below that are consistent with decompensated heart failure hemodynamics:

√ CO = 2.5 L/min	√ PCW = 30 mm Hg	
√ HR = 120 bpm	√ SVR = 1500 dyne·sec·cm^{-5}	
___ RA = 4 mm Hg	√ EF = 20%	

3. Patients with heart failure may have depressed oxygen consumption during exercise due to which of the following?
    a) decreased stroke volume

4. Each of the following is a phase of the cardiac cycle except:
    a) isovolumic diastole

5. An increase in vascular tone will lead to all of the following except:
    d) decreased systemic vascular resistance

6. Drugs may improve myocardial ischemia in failing hearts by:
    d) decreasing afterload to reduce myocardial oxygen consumption

7. The following are considered to be measureable "clinical" variables associated with heart failure except:
    b) vascular tone

8. Which of the following is not a measurable index of ventricular preload?
    b) systemic vascular resistance

9. Patients with heart failure typically have high vascular tone secondary to neurohormonal activation and chronic changes in vessel wall structure. This increase in vascular tone can result in which of the following?
    c) a greater increase in filling pressure with increased blood volume

Chapter 3 Quiz– Circulation Con't

10. All of the following contribute to the loss of control of the negative feedback loop in the neurohormonal activation of heart failure except:
    b) increased reservoirs of norepinephrine within post-synaptic sympathetic nerves

11. Long-term inotropic drug therapy can improve both quality of life and potential for long-term survival through significant increases in hemodynamic function in patients with heart failure.
    b) False

12. Chronic effects of reflex neurohormonal action (i.e., salt and water retention, vasocon- striction, and sympathetic stimulation) include:
    d) all of the above

13. The SOLVD trial showed that all of the following circulating neurohormones were associated with the progression of heart failure except:
    b) nitric oxide

Chapter 4 Quiz - Organ

1. Which of the following may contribute to the development of heart failure?
    e) all of the above

2. The total heart volume of the heart (i.e., myocardial solid plus chamber blood vol- umes) remains approximately the same at end-diastole and end-systole.
    a) True

3. As a mechanical pump, the heart operates within the limits imposed by end-systolic and diastolic ventricular pressure-volume relationships. A _____ spread between the two operating curves indicates a _____ performance of the heart as a pump.
    a) larger; better

4. As compared to systolic dysfunction, diastolic dysfunction is more commonly associ- ated with all of the following except:
    d) left ventricular dilatation

5. In the Frank-Starling ventricular performance curve, ventricular diastolic volume deter- mines ventricular _____ for systolic performance and diastolic pressure determines the potential for _____.
    b) preload; congestion

Chapter 4 Quiz - Organ Con't

6. Match the figure with the type of hypertrophy:
   a) normal heart
   b) concentric hypertrophy
   c) dilated hypertrophy

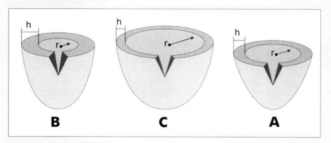

B   C   A

7. All of the following may contribute to decreased relaxation in diastolic dysfunction except:
   c) increased catecholamines

8. Factors which may lead to the spatial and temporal nonuniformity of load and contractility of the heart include all of the following except:
   b) valvular disease

Chapter 5 Quiz - Cell

1. Match the following myocyte component to its respective function:

c	myofibril
e	mitochondria
g	nucleus
d	sarcoplasmic reticulum
f	T-tubules
h	sarcolemma
a	lysosomes
b	sarcoplasm (cytoplasm)

   a. Intracellular digestion and proteolysis
   b. Provides cytosol in which rise and fall of ionized calcium occurs; contains other ions, small molecules, and proteins
   c. Interaction of thick and thin filaments during contraction cycle.
   d. Takes up and releases Ca^{++} during contraction cycle
   e. Provide high energy ATP chiefly for contraction and homeostasis
   f. Transmission of electrical signal from sarcolemma to cell interior
   g. mRNA synthesis
   h. Control of ionic gradients

Chapter 5 Quiz - Cell Con't

2. The heart functions as a circulatory pump by conversion of pressure-volume work to biochemical energy and the utilization of ATP by actin and myosin.
   b) False

3. Because of the LaPlace relationship, resting energy utilization per gram of heart tissue of the dilated failing heart is greater than the normal heart.
   a) True

4. Complete the following equation:

$$\frac{\text{ENERGY UTILIZATION}}{\text{GRAM OF HEART MUSCLE}} \quad \alpha \text{ SYSTOLIC WALL STRESS} \quad \cdot \quad \underline{\textbf{b) heart rate}}$$

5. Which of the following best describes the myocyte electromechanical interval?
   d) depolarization of electrical action potential $\rightarrow$ calcium release $\rightarrow$ force generation

6. What is the relationship between the level of calcium in the papillary muscle to the generation of force?
   c) $Ca^{++}\ \alpha$ Force

7. All of the following factors influence vascular smooth muscle cell contraction except:
   d) superoxide dismutase

8. Increasing the levels of intracellular c-AMP has which of the following effects on the cardiac and smooth muscles?
   b) increase in cardiac contractility and smooth muscle cell vasodilation

9. In heart failure, despite high levels of circulating norepinephrine, myocyte concentrations of c-AMP may be low because of a down regulation in the number and activity of cell membrane adrenergic β-receptors.
   a) True

Chapter 6 Quiz - Sarcomere

1. The myosin band of the sarcomere moves closer together during contraction and further apart during relaxation, while the Z lines remain constant throughout both processes.
   b) False

2. The myosin molecule orients its head toward the center of the sarcomere M line and its tail laterally. Aggregates of myosin molecules form a thick myofilament.
   b) False

CHAPTER 6 QUIZ - SARCOMERE CON'T

3. The myosin protein is composed of
   c) 6 subunits — 2 heavy and 4 light chains

4. All of the following is true of the troponin protein except:
   b) it fits into the grooves of the myosin thick filament

5. The action potential initiates the influx of calcium into the myocyte and the release of calcium from intracellular stores within the sarcoplasmic reticulum. Which of the following best describes the subsequent steps in the contractile process?
   d) binding of Ca^{++} to troponin C → conformational change in troponin trimer → displacement of tropomyosin → exposure of actin binding site → formation of actin-myosin crossbridge

6. All of the following events occur in the power stroke for muscle contraction except:
   a) No energy is required for calcium reuptake and muscle relaxation

CHAPTER 7 QUIZ -GENE

1. Heart size is a predictor of outcome in patients with heart failure.
   a) True

2. Which of the following are considered to be *triggers* of myocyte hypertrophy:
   d) all of the above

3. Which of the following is not involved in the pathway for activating transcription factors in cardiac muscle hypertrophy?
   a) angiotensin I

4. Apoptosis is an energy requiring process with characteristic fragmentation of chromosomal DNA which occurs usually without the presence of inflammatory cell infiltrates.
   a) True

5. Rats with heart failure have significantly _____ fibrosis fractional areas and _____ myocyte fractional areas compared to normal rats.
   b) greater; less

6. The myocyte is a source, rather than a target, for a spectrum of cytokines that depress heart function and contribute to ventricular enlargement.
   b) False

CHAPTER 8 QUIZ - MOLECULE

1. Which of the following has a dominant pattern of inheritance with variable penetrance?
    c) hypertrophic cardiomyopathy

2. All of the following are known genetic abnormalities that may lead to heart failure except:
    b) a frameshift mutation within the actin-myosin binding site

3. Patients with heart failure may have reduced synthesis of both the phospholamban as well as the calcium ATPase pump proteins which may reduce force generation with electrical depolarization.
    a) True

Case Scenario Solutions and Discussion

CHAPTER 9, SCENARIO SOLUTION #1

ASSESSMENT

Step 1 — Does the presentation fit a diagnosis of heart failure?

The physical exam findings of increased neck veins indicate an increased venous pressure suggestive of increased right heart filling pressures. In addition, bibasilar rales indicates pulmonary congestion. The presentation, therefore, fits a diagnosis of heart failure. An echocardiogram is indicated to demonstrate cardiovascular causes of the patient's presenation.

Step 2 — Is LV function abnormal?

Echocardiogram finding of an ejection fraction of 20% identifies systolic dysfunction. The four chamber enlargement of this patient's heart demonstrates that this patient has a chronic cardiac condition since it takes time for the heart structure to remodel in this way.

Step 3 — Are there treatable causes? (Recommendations)

The etiology of this patient's heart failure, although probably non-ischemic cardiomyopathy, is unknown. An Adenosine ^{99m}Tc-sestamibi stress test will screen the patient for myocardial ischemia. I would not recommend Swan-Ganz catheterization since this patient should respond to clinically guided empiric treatment. Cardiac catheterization is not mandatory at this time since there is no overt evidence of coronary disease. An endomyocardial biopsy is unlikely to yield evidence of treatable conditions of the heart that would be identified by histologic evaluation of myocardial tissue. A V/Q scan is not necessary since there is no predominance of right heart failure.

Question 1a

a) Adenosine ^{99m}Tc-sestamibi stress test

☑ *Patients with heart failure usually have an abnormal ECG, chest x-ray, or both.*

Step 2 and Step 3 Revisited with Echo-Doppler Variations

The finding of asymmetric septal hypertrophy on echocardiogram leads to the diagnosis of idiopathic hypertrophic subaortic stenosis (IHSS) — a genetically based hypertrophic cardiomyopathy. Further testing is unnecessary; I would treat this patient with β-blockers and cautiously administer diuretics.

Question 1b

f) none of the above

Concentric hypertrophy and diastolic dysfunction found by echo-Doppler are consistent with hypertensive heart disease. The Doppler finding of E-A reversal indicates that there is a decrease in early filling of the left ventricle and a compensatory increase in filling following atrial contraction. I would screen this patient for coronary disease using an adenosine ^{99m}Tc-sestamibi stress test and treat her with diuretics and ACE inhibitors. Alternatively, β-blockers could be substituted for ACE inhibitors to control this patient's hypertension and possibly improve diastolic filling by slowing heart rate.

Question 1c

a) adenosine ^{99m}Tc-sestamibi stress test

Echo-Doppler suggests diastolic dysfunction of the LV. The dilated and hypokinetic RV suggests systolic dysfunction due to increased afterload of this chamber, specifically either Cor Pulmonale and/or pulmonary emboli. A V/Q scan would test this hypothesis. Diuretics will help reduce systemic congestion.

Question 1d

f) V/Q scan

The sclerocalcific changes in the aortic valve with decreased cusp separation indicate aortic stenosis. A cardiac catheterization would assess heart function and exclude associated coronary artery disease prior to aortic valve replacement which could reverse findings of heart failure after surgery.

Question 1d

c) Cardiac catheterization

☑ *Clinical strategy for the same patient varies with differing echo-doppler findings.*

Chapter 9, Scenario Solution #2

Step 1 — Does the presentation fit a diagnosis of heart failure?

This patient's increased neck veins suggest an increased right heart filling pressure. On physical exam, the bibasilar rales suggests pulmonary congestion. Diabetes mellitus is a risk factor for CAD. Patients with this condition are also at risk for "silent ischemia" since they may have a sensory neuropathy of internal organs including the heart. Diabetes may also be associated with a non-ischemic cardiomyopathy, therefore, indicating further cardiovascular assessment.

Step 2 — Is LV function abnormal?

Although LV systolic function is found to be normal, is it important to identify treatable causes of diastolic function.

Step 3 — Are there treatable causes? (Recommendations)

I would recommend a cardiac catheterization for this patient to screen for CAD. An Adenosine ^{99m}Tc-sestamibi stress test could be an initial screening test for CAD, but could yield a false negative result in the presence of three vessel disease and global myocardial ischemia.

Question 2

c) Cardiac catheterization

Chapter 9, Scenario Solution #3

Step 1 — Does the presentation fit a diagnosis of heart failure?

Increased neck veins indicate increased right heart filling pressures due to an increased venous pressure. Bibasilar rales as well as the increased interstitial pattern on chest x-ray suggest pulmonary congestion.

Step 2 — Is LV function abnormal?

An ejection fraction greater than 50% with concentric hypertrophy is consistent with diastolic dysfunction.

Step 3 — Are there treatable causes? (Recommendations)

On echo, the speckled pattern is consistent with an infiltration of amyloid protein; urinalysis showing 3+ protein also

Question 3

e) Endomyocardial biopsy

supports amyloidosis with kidney involvement. In addition, free wall hypertrophy of the right ventricle is consistent with infiltrative cardiomyopathy or hypertrophy due to pulmonary hypertension. Biopsy showing evidence of amyloidosis would confirm the diagnosis and potentially focus patient therapy.

CHAPTER 10, SCENARIO SOLUTION #1

KEY CLINICAL FINDINGS

This patient's history of ischemic cardiomyopathy suggests long-standing ischemic heart disease and impaired ventricular function. On physical exam, there is no indication of increased venous pressure or pulmonary congestion. This patient's asthma could be a contraindication to β-blockers. Lisinopril is being used to blunt disease progression.

THERAPUTIC STRATEGY

Digoxin should reduce this patient's likelihood of hospitalization due to worsening heart failure, but will not affect overall mortality. I would avoid carvedilol in this case because this drug could exacerbate the patient's asthma.

Although there is no contraindication to losartan, isosorbide dinitrate and hydralazine, or amlodipine there is less evidence that this would improve symptoms or disease progression when added to an ACE inhibitor.

Question 1

c) digoxin

CHAPTER 10, SCENARIO SOLUTION #2

KEY CLINICAL FINDINGS

The finding of stable fatigue on climbing one flight of stairs is consistent with a history of NYHA Class II-III heart failure. Trace edema is present but right heart filling pressures are not high since the neck veins are not distended. Venous stasis may be the cause.

Question 2

e) carvedilol

☑ *This patient can benefit from effective neurohormonal management to blunt disease progression.*

THERAPUTIC STRATEGY

In addition to this patient's lisinopril, digoxin, furosemide, and potassium, I would add carvedilol to further reduce disease progression. Carvedilol should not be used in patients who have symptoms at rest because β-blockade may lead to acute worsening of hemodynamic function.

At this time, the indication for amiodarone would only be for atrial or ventricular arrhythmias. Although there is no contraindication to losartan, isosorbide dinitrate and hydralazine, or amlodipine there is less evidence that this would improve symptoms or disease progression when added to an ACE inhibitor.

CHAPTER 10, SCENARIO SOLUTION #3

KEY CLINICAL FINDINGS

Increased creatinine suggests impaired intrinsic kidney function or reduced renal perfusion.

Question 3

b) isosorbide dinitrate & hydralazine

THERAPUTIC STRATEGY

Therapy for this patient would include either adding the combination of isosorbide dinitrate and hydralazine to the ACE inhibitor that he is currently taking, or substituting this combination for lisinopril to improve Class IV symptoms. If symptoms improved, he would potentially be a candidate for carvedilol to reduce disease progression. I would continue furosemide to reduce edema.

At this time, the indication for amiodarone would only be for atrial or ventricular arrhythmias. Although there is no contraindication to losartan or amlodipine there is less evidence that this would improve symptoms or disease progression when added to an ACE inhibitor.

☑ *Patients who are intolerant of ACE inhibitors or have persistent hypertension despite ACE inhibition and β-blockade may benefit from ARBs.*

CHAPTER 10, SCENARIO SOLUTION #4

KEY CLINICAL FINDINGS

This patient's blood pressure is elevated but she does not appear to have systemic congestion.

THERAPUTIC STRATEGY

Data from the PRAISE trial suggests that amlodipine may improve survival in patients with non-ischemic cardiomyopathy. This drug would reduce this patient's blood pressure. Isosorbide dinitrate and hydralazine may also help symptoms.

At this time, the indication for amiodarone would only be for atrial or ventricular arrhythmias. Presently, this patient's condition is not consistent with a need for anticoagulation. Although there is no contraindication to losartan or isosorbide dinitrate and hydralazine, there is less evidence that this would improve symptoms or disease progression when added to an ACE inhibitor.

Question 4

d) amlodipine

CHAPTER 10, SCENARIO SOLUTION #5

KEY CLINICAL FINDINGS

This patient's cough may be due to an intolerance of ACE inhibitors. Flat neck veins suggest, but do not prove that her cough is not due to pulmonary congestion.

THERAPUTIC STRATEGY

I would take this patient off lisinopril since she appears to have an intolerance to ACE inhibitors and would start her on losartan so she can continue to benefit from the effects of angiotensin II blockade. There is no evidence of pulmonary congestion on examination. I would attempt to further exclude this as a reason for cough by obtaining a chest x-ray. I would continue furosemide to reduce edema.

At this time, the indication for amiodarone would only be for atrial or ventricular arrhythmias. Although there is no contraindication to isosorbide dinitrate and hydralazine or amlodipine there is less evidence that this would improve symptoms or disease progression when added to an ACE inhibitor.

Question 5

a) losartan

Chapter 11, Scenario Solution #1

Key Clinical Findings

Since this patient recently was pregnant, it is possible that she has peripartum cardiomyopathy. Cardiomegaly and pulmonary congestion also support this diagnosis.

Question 1a

a) Right heart catheterization

Question 1b

Evaluate the therapies listed below for this inpatient:

a. Very helpful
b. Marginally helpful
c. Not helpful or potentially harmful

___b___ 1. nitroprusside

___b___ 2. nitroglycerin SL

___b___ 3. nitroglycerin IV

___b___ 4. nitroglycerin topical

___b___ 5. dopamine

___c___ 6. amlodipine

___c___ 7. β-blocker

___a___ 8. milrinone

___b___ 9. ACE Inhibitor

___c___ 10. amiodarone

Discharge Summary

The patient was given milrinone and her hemodynamics improved (right). Milrinone was weaned once the patient was afebrile. Cultures were negative. Diagnosis: Peripartum cardiomyopathy, viral syndrome. Patient was discharged on digoxin, furosemide, lisinopril, and potassium. β-blockers were to be started as an outpatient.

Hemodynamics on Milrinone

BP = 100/68
HR = 110
RA = 8
PA = 26/14
PCW = 13
Cardiac Index = 2.2 L/min/m²

CHAPTER 11, SCENARIO SOLUTION #2

RECOMMENDATIONS 2a

This patient is suffering from cardiogenic shock and profound hypotension. This patient would benefit from an IABP to decrease afterload and increase coronary diastolic perfusion. If necessary, IV epinephrine could be used while this patient is emergently transported to the catheterization lab for a PTCA/stent procedure since high doses of dopamine are already being used. IV thrombolysis could be used if the hospital facility does not have a catheterization lab. Neither IV milrinone nor IV nitroglycerin should be used since both of these agents can decrease blood pressure.

Question 2a

c) IABP and cardiac catheterization

RECOMMENDATIONS 2b

This patient could receive IV epinephrine to maintain blood pressure until placement of ECLS. Placement of ECLS will allow reperfusion therapy to be performed.

Question 2b

c) Placement of percutaneous extracorporeal life support (ECLS)

☑ *For cardiogenic shock, 0.1 – 1.0 mg boluses of IV epinephrine can temporarily maintain the circulation until mechanical support can be initiated.*

RECOMMENDATIONS 2c

ECLS could be withdrawn after the cardiac function improves. Subsequently, dopamine and/or IABP could be resumed to allow weaning from ECLS. This patient has already been percutaneously revascularized and is still a poor candidate for bypass surgery. Placement of a left ventricular assist device, if necessary, could be considered if the patient was approved for heart transplant.

Question 2c

a) Continue ECLS support

DISCHARGE SUMMARY

On the second hospital day, dopamine was resumed, IABP was reinitiated, and ECLS was removed in the operating room. Subsequently, the patient recovered without neurologic deficit and was ambulated. Nineteen days after presentation, radionuclide ejection fraction was measured at 32%.

Index

Heart Failure Online

www.heartfailure.org

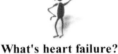

What's heart failure?

How the heart works

Do I have heart failure?

Frequently asked
questions

Living with heart
failure

Links to related sites

The webmasters

What's new?

The website dedicated to the patient with heart failure.

Sponsored in part by the Sharp Foundation for
Cardiovascular Research and Education
and the San Diego Cardiac Center.